THE
PREGNANCY
PRESCRIPTION

The
Success-Oriented
Approach to
Overcoming Infertility

Hugh D. Melnick, MD
and
Nancy Intrator

The Josara Companies, Inc.

The treatment plan described in this book has been developed based on the accumulated training, experience, research, and opinion of the authors. However, because each patient is unique, readers are urged to consult with a qualified physician before embarking on any elements of the course of treatment described herein. The author and publisher are not responsible for any adverse consequences resulting from the various forms of treatment described in this book.

Publisher's Cataloging-in-Publication
(Provided by Quality Books, Inc.)

Melnick, Hugh D.

The pregnancy prescription: the success-oriented approach to overcoming infertility / Hugh D. Melnick and Nancy Intrator. — 1 st ed.

p. cm.

Includes index.
Preassigned LCCN: 97-94304
ISBN: 0-9660419-0-9

1. Infertility—Popular works. 2. Human reproductive technology —Popularworks. I. Intrator, Nancy. II. Title.

RG201.M45 1998   618.1'78
                           QBI97-2 1 79

Library of Congress Catalog Card Number: 97-94304

ISBN Number: 0-9660419-0-9

Additional copies of *The Pregnancy Prescription* can be purchased from The Josara Companies, Inc., c/o Pathway Book Services, 4 White Brook Rd., Gilsum, NH 03448, or by calling 800-345-6665. Special discounts are available for quantity sales.

become pregnant. The doctor might perform a second HSG to make sure her tubes hadn't closed up again, or he might order additional tests both for her (an endometrial biopsy) and for Mark (hamster egg penetration test). None of these tests would reveal what was preventing the pregnancy.

Finally, the doctor might throw up his hands and suggest that the couple try IVF as a last resort. As we saw in the previous example, IVF would ultimately prove successful in making Susan pregnant. Why? Because in addition to blocking off the distal (outer) end of one of her Fallopian tubes, Susan's infection had also caused subtle damage to the insides of both tubes. The damage was both *undetectable and untreatable.* So although the surgery eliminated Susan's most obvious physical problem, she was still incapable of conceiving naturally. IVF offered her only chance for a pregnancy.

Kate and Steven—The Success-Oriented Approach

Kate, an artist, and Steven, a writer, had been trying for a pregnancy for almost 2 years. Since Kate was only 31-years-old, the couple was reluctant to consult a fertility specialist, but since they both wanted a big family, they decided that it would be wise not to wait too long before seeking help.

Neither case history indicated any problem, and Kate's hysterosalpingogram and blood tests were normal. However, Steven's semen analysis showed his sperm to have marginally abnormal morphology (shape) and motility (movement). A physical exam revealed him to be suffering from a varicocele (varicose vein of the testes).

The doctor recommended a diagnostic IVF cycle to see if Steven's sperm were capable of fertilizing Kate's eggs. Thanks to medication, Kate produced 12 eggs, which the embryologist divided into two groups. He exposed the first group to Steven's sperm in the normal manner to see if they could fertilize naturally and performed ICSI (injection of a single sperm directly into the egg) with the eggs in the second group. Two of the eggs in the first group fertilized, as did five from the ICSI group. Unfortunately, none of the four embryos that were transferred back to Kate's uterus implanted; neither did the remaining three embryos, which had been frozen and then thawed and transferred into her uterus during a subsequent cycle.

For their next IVF cycle, Kate was able to produce only nine eggs. Thanks to ICSI, Seven's sperm successfully fertilized six of the eggs *in vitro*. The couple elected to transfer all six embryos back into Kate's uterus. Several weeks later, Kate learned she was pregnant with twins.

Steven's varicocele and marginally abnormal sperm had appeared to be the obvious cause of this couple's infertility. But the initial IVF trial demonstrated that, even unassisted, Steven's sperm were capable of fertilizing some of Kate's eggs, but at a lower percentage rate than normal. Their inability to conceive was caused by this reduced fertilization rate combined with some undiagnosable factor in Kate that was successfully bypassed by the IVF procedure.

Kate and Steven—The Diagnosis-Oriented Approach

As soon as a diagnosis-oriented physician would have become aware of Steven's sperm abnormalities (abnormal shape and movement), he would have suspected a varicocele. When the physical exam confirmed his suspicions, the doctor would have recommended that Steven undergo surgery to correct the problem—especially since the results of the couple's complete diagnostic workup would have revealed no other problems that could be causing their infertility.

The operation, though not serious, would have caused Steven some discomfort for several weeks. A post-surgical semen analysis would probably have demonstrated some improvement in his sperm's motility and morphology, but the change would not be dramatic.

One year later, Kate still would not have become pregnant. The doctor would probably have advised the couple to try fertility drugs combined with intrauterine insemination, since he could find no treatable cause for their continued inability to conceive. He would advise them to proceed to IVF only after it had become clear that the IUI was not succeeding.

POTENTIAL PITFALLS OF THE DIAGNOSIS-ORIENTED APPROACH

As seen with both couples, a problem with the diagnosis-oriented approach is that many of the diagnostic techniques and procedures traditionally used to treat infertility can be expensive, unreliable, invasive, and time consuming. This is an especially important consideration for women in their mid-to-late thirties and early forties, who may be nearing the end of their reproductive years.

But perhaps more important, the case studies illustrate that many of the factors responsible for causing infertility are impossible to diagnose and/or treat by any method. The American Society for Reproductive Medicine estimates that fewer than half of all infertile couples can be helped by techniques such as fertility drugs, simple inseminations, and surgery. In addition, there may be more than one factor preventing the couple from conceiving. It may be possible to "cure" one problem, but other undiagnosed factors could still make unassisted conception impossible.

The reality is that the process of conception is too complex to allow for the diagnosis and treatment of all the potential factors that may be causing a couple's infertility. There are simply too many steps at which problems may occur, both at the microscopic and genetic level. Only the most obvious causes can be accurately diagnosed and resolved.

SO WHY ISN'T EVERYONE SUCCESS-ORIENTED?

In general, the success-oriented strategy hasn't been universally adopted because of its reliance on the advanced reproductive techniques, such as IVF. There are a number of reasons why some doctors and potential patients are uncomfortable with these procedures.

Newness

Although infertility has been around since biblical times, the assisted reproductive techniques like IVF are still relatively new. In fact, the world's first IVF baby was just born in 1978. People are naturally slow to accept new ways of doing things— and doctors are no exception. Both doctors and patients are likely to be uninformed as to the potential value of these techniques for diagnostic as well as treatment purposes.

Lack of Awareness

There is a general lack of awareness of how much progress has been made in advanced reproductive technology and just how accessible these options have become. IVF is no longer an invasive procedure requiring surgery or even general anesthesia, and variations on the basic IVF procedure have dramatically increased its potential for helping infertile couples conceive. For example, by employing intracytoplasmic sperm injection (ICSI), a single sperm can be injected directly into an egg to make it fertilize, making fatherhood possible even for men with extremely low sperm counts or misshapen sperm.

Misinformation Regarding Safety

A number of stories and articles have implied that the medications used in IVF may increase a woman's chances of developing certain cancers. What the public may not realize is that many experts consider the study on which that charge was based to have been both poorly designed and irrelevant——especially since most patients in the study took clomiphene citrate, a drug which is not normally used in IVF. Better-designed studies and years of clinical experience with the drugs that *are* used in IVF have not shown any association with an increased risk of cancer.

Confusing Success Rates

There is wide variation between IVF centers in terms of success rates. At this point, neither doctors nor interested patients are adept at interpreting these differences and evaluating the various options.

Cost Misperceptions

IVF is perceived as being outrageously expensive. However, although the average cost of an IVF procedure in the United States is $7,800, this figure can vary significantly according to geographic location and the number of procedures the clinic performs per year. And since using IVF as an early stage diagnostic and treatment tool can eliminate the need for many of the traditional fertility tests and procedures, IVF can actually help reduce the total cost of infertility treatment.

SUMMARY

By eliminating the time and expense associated with extensive diagnostic testing and treatments, the success-oriented approach can expand the power of nature and help many couples conceive more quickly and cost-effectively. When used as an element in the success-oriented approach to infertility treatment, IVF is a valuable diagnostic and treatment tool that can help identify the source of a couple's problem, bypass the most likely problem areas, and offer at least a 20 percent chance of conception each time it is performed.

C H A P T E R   4

STEP 1:

The Streamlined Workup

No matter which approach to infertility treatment you select, the first step will probably be for you and your partner to undergo some sort of diagnostic workup. This workup can be as brief as having the doctor simply ask you a few questions, or as extensive as to actually involve surgery. The number of tests you are advised to undergo and the amount of time you spend on testing, rather than treatment, will largely depend on whether your doctor follows a diagnosis- or success-oriented approach to infertility treatment.

Even if your doctor advises only a few of the most basic infertility tests, you still may find some portions of the workup embarrassing, or feel that your privacy is being invaded. You will probably need to answer detailed questions about your sexual practices. Women may find themselves lying on the exam table with their legs spread more often than they would have ever thought possible. Their partners will probably become adept at ejaculating into sterile containers.

Distasteful as all this may be, don't let shyness deter you from your ultimate goal of conceiving a child. Your doctor and the rest of the office staff should try to make you as comfortable as possible with what they need to do, and they should be scrupulous about protecting your privacy and keeping your secrets. Also, though this may all be new to you, this is what the doctors and nurses do every day. Finally, bear in mind that with a success-oriented physician, you may need to undergo far less testing than with those who follow the diagnosis-and-treatment approach.

THE DIAGNOSIS-ORIENTED WORKUP

Diagnosis-oriented fertility specialists use tests and procedures to try to determine exactly which parts of the reproductive systems aren't working correctly. Their meticulous and exhaustive testing will include many—if not all—of the following:

The Diagnosis-Oriented Workup For Her:

- Patient history

- Physical exam

- Cervical cultures to test for current infection by chlamydia or mycoplasma

- Blood tests for hormone levels

- Ovulation tests via basal body temperature reporting or at-home urine testing kits

- Pelvic sonogram

- At least one hysterosalpingogram (HSG): a dye-assisted x-ray of the woman's reproductive organs

- At least one post-coital test (PCT): after the couple has intercourse, the doctor examines the woman's cervical mucus under a microscope to evaluate whether her partner's sperm can function inside of her

- An endometrial biopsy: the doctor removes a sample of the woman's uterine lining and sends it to a pathologist for analysis

- At least one diagnostic/therapeutic laparoscopy: a surgical procedure that allows the doctor to view the woman's internal organs

The Diagnosis-Oriented Workup For Him:

- Patient history

- Physical exam

- At least one semen analysis

- A hamster test: to see whether the sperm is able to penetrate a hamster egg

- Other indirect tests of sperm function

The Diagnosis-Oriented Workup For Both:

- Anti-sperm antibody blood tests to determine if either partner is producing substances that may block fertilization of an egg

THE SUCCESS-ORIENTED WORKUP

Success-oriented doctors only need to learn enough from the workup to be able to determine which form of treatment would make the best starting point. They tend to rely on only a few rapid, basic, non-invasive tests to rule out major and obvious problems. This is because success-oriented physicians believe that the majority of disorders that cause infertility are impossible to accurately diagnose. These doctors have found that the ability to use IVF early on in the process has eliminated some potential diagnostic errors which may result from the traditional workup. For success-oriented infertility specialists, IVF is the ultimate diagnostic procedure.

The success-oriented, streamlined workup can save you precious time (the complete battery of standard infertility tests can take up to a year, or more), pain (some standard diagnostic tests involve surgery), and substantially reduce the costs normally associated with the traditional diagnostic process.

The Success-Oriented Workup For Her
Patient history

Health and reproductive histories are important elements of the streamlined workup. The information provided during a history can help the doctor decide whether the couple should proceed directly to an IVF trial or if other tests and/or procedures should be performed first.

Age

First and foremost, the doctor needs to know the patient's age. In general, the younger the woman, the better her chances for conceiving, since the quality of a woman's eggs tend to decline as she gets older. For example, if a 37- to 42-year-old woman has been able to easily conceive in the past, but her two most recent conceptions ended in early miscarriage, it would be reasonable to assume that her eggs have been adversely affected by her age. The doctor would probably perform some hormonal tests to verify this hypothesis; however, such a patient could prove infertile even despite fairly normal test values.

Medical history

Since certain diseases, such as rheumatoid arthritis, may affect a woman's ability to maintain a pregnancy, the doctor needs to know the patient's complete medical history. Information about her menstrual periods—their regularity, duration, heaviness of flow, etc.—as well as any previous gynecologic infections and/or surgery is also vital. It is particularly important to know if a patient has had any abortions, since any surgical procedure, whether major or minor, may result in subtle, undetectable tubal damage or in the formation of internal scar tissue.

Reproductive history

Another important piece of information for the doctor is whether the patient has ever been pregnant. A previous pregnancy is usually considered a good sign, since this suggests that the woman's egg supply is of good genetic quality. But if a woman with a normal menstrual history and patent (open) tubes admits that she has never conceived despite unprotected intercourse with several partners over a period of years, there's a chance that her eggs are defective in some way. Or, she may be producing a subtle "blocking" factor (a totally unidentifiable substance that is preventing her eggs from being able to fertilize in her body). An IVF trial gives the physician a chance to determine which is the more likely cause of her failure to conceive.

Pelvic sonogram

A pelvic sonogram is the most important "examination" that can be performed on infertile women. To perform the sonogram, the technician or physician inserts a small probe that is shaped like a wand into the woman's vagina. Although some women find the procedure a little embarrassing the first few times it is performed, vaginal ultrasound is completely painless. And unlike abdominal sonograms, this exam does not require the patient to have a full bladder.

The sonographic image projected onto the screen shows the size and shape of the uterus and endometrial cavity, the presence and position of the ovaries and whether there is a reserve of eggs present in the ovaries. A sonogram can detect abnormalities in the uterus and ovaries and show the doctor if the Fallopian tubes are swollen or filled with fluid (hydrosalpinx), which means that they were probably blocked as a result of a prior tubal infection. It can also detect endometrial cysts on the ovaries, which can adversely affect egg production.

Test for infection

Although vaginal infections do not cause infertility, pelvic infections caused by certain organisms, such as chlamydia, can cause irreparable damage to the Fallopian tubes and prevent a woman from being able to conceive naturally. This can happen in one of two ways: either the tubes become occluded (blocked) as a result of an inflammatory response to the infection, or the tubal lining becomes damaged, thus interfering with its ability to propel the oocyte (egg) or embryo towards the uterus.

Since chlamydia infections do not always cause symptoms, a woman may not know if she has ever had one. The only way to be absolutely sure is to test her blood for the presence of the anti-chlamydial antibody. If the test results are positive, it means that she may have been infected with chlamydia at least once in the past. And if she has been unable to become pregnant despite tubes that appear to be open, the infection may have caused some undetectable damage to the lining of her Fallopian tubes. It is likely that such women will need to use IVF to bypass their tubes in order to become pregnant.

Mycoplasma, another organism that has been implicated as a possible cause of infertility and miscarriage, can be difficult to detect via a culture. Because of this, somewhere during their infertility treatment it may be useful for both the male and the female to have simultaneous treatment with an antibiotic such as Vibramycin™ (doxycycline: a tetracycline derivative), which has proven effective against the organism. Some data suggest that this treatment may increase the chances for pregnancy. Side effects of the medication may include diarrhea, yeast infections, and photosensitivity; to offset these effects, patients taking Vibramycin should eat yogurt and stay out of direct sunlight.

Hormone level testing

Although the quality of a woman's eggs usually declines as she becomes older, chronological age is not always the best way to assess a woman's potential fertility. Hormone level testing cannot always help to predict which women *will* be able to conceive. However, elevated levels of certain hormones can be reliable indicators of which women will be *unable* to achieve a pregnancy.

Follicle Stimulating Hormone (FSH)

As the name suggests, this is the hormone that signals the ovaries to begin producing an egg for a new cycle. Testing a woman's FSH level on day 2 to 3 of her menstrual cycle provides the best indication of how well she will respond to fertility drugs—a measure that correlates with her overall chances for becoming pregnant. Again, the test suggests whether pregnancy *cannot* occur more closely than whether it can. In general, the lower a woman's FSH on day 2 to 3 of her cycle, the better.

FSH	CHANCES FOR PREGNANCY
<12 mlU/mL	best chances for pregnancy
12-15 mlU/mL	may not respond well to ovarian stimulation
15-20 mlU/mL	depleted pool of eggs; reduced chances for pregnancy
20-25 mlU/mL	may ovulate, but prognosis for pregnancy is poor
>25 mlU/mL	will probably not become pregnant without donor eggs

Since FSH levels fluctuate on a monthly basis, the day 2 to 3 FSH level predicts a woman's ovulation response *for that particular cycle only.* For example, if a 40-year-old has an FSH of 19 on day 3, she will probably not respond well to fertility drugs that month, and it would be wise to stop treatment for that particular cycle. During her next cycle, however, her day 3 FSH may go down to 12, and she may be better able to respond to the medication. Unfortunately, once a woman has been shown to have a high FSH level, her chances for becoming pregnant are greatly reduced—even though she may occasionally produce numerous eggs in response to fertility drugs. An exception is the younger (28- to 35-year-old) woman who may be able to become pregnant despite an occasional "high FSH" month.

Estradiol (Estrogen)

A woman's estradiol level on day 2 to 3 of her cycle is another important predictor of her potential fertility. If her estradiol level on day 2 to 3 is greater than 80 mg/ml, she may be having abnormal follicle production—-similar, in pattern, to early pre-menopause. This is not a good sign for the woman who wants to become pregnant.

Prolactin

Elevated prolactin (the hormone that stimulates milk secretion) levels can interfere with the doctor's ability to induce ovulation in some patients, while others remain able to ovulate quite normally. This is because a woman can secrete any of five varieties of the prolactin hormone molecule. Although the blood test will detect elevated levels of any of these five varieties, only one or two actually affect the menstrual cycle. Elevated levels of the others may cause certain physical effects (e.g., the production of fluid from the nipples), but since they do not inhibit or block ovulation, they do not need to be treated. Women with prolactin levels that are consistently elevated should have a CAT scan or MRI study of their pituitary gland to determine whether a small, benign growth is causing the excess prolactin production.

Thyroid

From the 1940s to1960s many infertile women and women with miscarriages were treated with thyroid medication. We now know that primary infertility is rarely caused by thyroid disturbance, and such treatment is unnecessary. Only extreme cases of hypothyroidism (underactive thyroid) will disrupt the menstrual cycle and cause a woman to stop getting her period. If a woman with an underactive thyroid does succeed in becoming pregnant, her fetus may be adversely affected unless she takes supplemental thyroid hormone. Hyperthyroidism (overactive thyroid) can be a medical emergency and must be treated promptly. The usual symptoms are very heavy menstrual periods, weight loss, nervousness, heart palpitations, and sweating.

Ovulation tests

Today, the best way to accurately assess whether or not ovulation is taking place is via vaginal ultrasound. The more traditional methods of detecting and/or predicting ovulation, i.e., measurement of a woman's basal body temperature (BBT) or urine testing for LH, can be time-consuming, may provide inconsistent results, and are generally unreliable.

By examining the woman via sonogram at various times during her menstrual cycle, the doctor can directly tell whether or not the patient is producing follicles (each of which presumably contains an egg) and if they are able to be released from the ovaries. For example, if a woman has a 30-day cycle, a sonogram performed on day 14 or 15 should show a mature, 20 mm follicle in the ovary. A follow-up sonogram performed 48 hours later should show that the follicle has burst and that the egg has been released. The doctor can also use the sonogram to see whether the woman's endometrium (uterine lining) is developing normally over the course of her menstrual cycle.

Hysterosalpingogram (HSG)

Since blocked Fallopian tubes are responsible for preventing pregnancy in up to 30 percent of infertile couples, the next step in the workup would probably be a hysterosalpingogram (HSG), a special kind of x-ray that is 85 to 90 percent accurate in diagnosing tubal blockages. The HSG can also diagnose a hydrosalpinx (fluid in the tubes).

To perform the HSG, the doctor injects a dye through the woman's cervix and into her uterus and Fallopian tubes. A series of x-ray pictures of the pelvic region is taken as the dye is being injected. If the woman's tubes are open, the x-rays will show the dye flowing freely out of the ends and into the woman's abdominal cavity, where it will be absorbed. If the dye cannot flow freely, it means that the tube is blocked.

Although the HSG itself is painless, the woman will probably feel a sense of pressure as the dye is injected. The dye injection may also cause some cramping or mild pain. This generally subsides soon after the procedure has been completed, but over-the-counter pain relievers such as Advil™ or other non-steroidal anti-inflammatory drugs taken 1 to 2 hours before the procedure can help prevent most of the discomfort.

Women with iodine (shellfish) allergies will also be allergic to the dye used in the HSG. For these patients, the doctor might utilize ultrasound, injecting the tubes with saline (salt-water) instead of the dye to visually check whether the Fallopian tubes are open.

What the x-ray may not show
Even if the HSG shows the woman's tubes as appearing to be open, they may still not function normally. There is no test—not even the insertion of a small telescope (Falloposcope) into the tubes—that can show how well the tubes perform. Therefore, it is important not to rule out the possibility of tubal damage as a cause of a woman's infertility despite the presence of a normal HSG.

If the HSG shows that fluid has accumulated in the Fallopian tube, the condition is called a hydrosalpinx. The blockage usually occurs at the far, fimbriated end of the Fallopian tube, which becomes sealed shut as a result of scar tissue formation. Most often, a hydrosalpinx results from a prior chlamydial or other bacterial infection, and the patient may have a positive anti-chlamydial antibody blood test. The fluid that accumulates in the tube contains no active bacteria or viruses, but it does contain many protein substances. The presence of a hydrosalpinx indicates that the tubal lining, which is vital to the fertilization process, is irrevocably damaged.

A significant number of women will conceive after the HSG if oil-based (rather than water-based) dye solution is used. Some theories suggest that the pressure of the thick solution may mechanically "flush-out" the tubes. It is our theory that the oil-based dye attracts the scavenger cells in the woman's immune system. This temporarily diverts them from being attracted to and attacking the sperm and egg, thereby allowing conception to take place in some patients.

Post-Coital Test

The Post-Coital Test (PCT) provides information as to whether the male's sperm are able to reach and survive in the female's cervical mucus. For the PCT, a couple is instructed to have intercourse around the time of ovulation, when the mucus is most copious. The woman is then asked to visit the doctor's office 12 to 24 hours afterward so that a sample of her mucus can be observed under the microscope. The test isn't painful, and the embarrassment a woman may feel at having her sexual activity so openly documented will probably be offset by the wonder of being able to watch her partner's sperm swimming around under the microscope!

By examining and counting the sperm in the sample, the doctor can tell whether the male's sperm can survive in his partner's cervical mucus and whether they are strong enough to make it through the vagina and cervical canal to enter the uterus and tubes. But like any diagnostic test for infertility, the PCT is far from infallible. Pregnancies have been reported in cycles in which there has been a poor PCT, with no sperm found in the woman's mucus at the time of ovulation.

The Success-Oriented Workup For Him

The recent development of Intracytoplasmic Sperm Injection (ICSI), a procedure in which a single sperm is injected directly into the egg to cause fertilization, has revolutionized the diagnosis and treatment of male infertility and eliminated the need for most of the traditional fertility tests and procedures for men. With the success-oriented approach, only a few tests remain necessary for the male.

Patient history

The health and reproductive history can help the doctor determine whether or not the couple should begin with the earlier steps in *The Pregnancy Prescription* or proceed directly to IVF, and whether ICSI should be employed.

The most important element of the male's history is whether he has created a pregnancy—either naturally or via IVF—during the past ten years. If so, this strongly implies that his sperm, no matter what the count, should be biologically capable of fertilizing an egg. This may not be true of a man who has had a vasectomy reversal in the intervening years since the pregnancy, since in some cases, post-vasectomy sperm may not be able to achieve fertilization normally.

Another signal that there may be a potential problem with the sperm supply is a history of undescended testes, or diseases such as mumps, epididymitis (infection of the epididymis), or prostatitis (infection of the prostate gland). Past exposure to such harmful substances as lead, cigarette smoke, marijuana, or excessive alcohol may also adversely affect sperm in some men, but there are no observable ill-effects in many others.

Semen analysis

Traditionally, the semen analysis has been the key diagnostic exam for men. For this test, the male is asked to ejaculate into a sterile container—usually while he is in the doctor's office or lab. Men who feel too inhibited to be able to bring themselves to orgasm in such a foreign environment should be permitted to produce the specimen off-site, as long as they bring it to the doctor's office in the specified time period, keep the sample at room temperature, and follow all other instructions. Within 1-2 hours of receiving the specimen, a computerized semen analysis can provide information as to the quantity of living, moving sperm, motility (movement), velocity (speed), and morphology (shape) of the man's sperm.

Unfortunately, semen analysis has proven disappointing in differentiating between which men can produce a pregnancy and which cannot, since many men with poor quality sperm do succeed in fathering children naturally. In reality, no particular parameter in the sperm count can truly provide an accurate indication of the male's fertility—with the possible exception of velocity, which we have found to be an accurate predictor of the sperm's potential ability to fertilize an egg. If, after processing and incubation, the male's sperm are found to swim slower than 60 microns per second, it has been our experience that the sperm will be unable to fertilize an egg on their own and the embryologist will need to perform ICSI to achieve fertilization for that couple.

The Success-Oriented Workup For Both
In vitro Fertilization

As a diagnostic test, *IVF provides the doctor with the most accurate indication of where the reproductive process is going awry.* For example, if a couple fails to conceive through intercourse or intrauterine insemination and the woman has one or more diagnosed fertility problems (e.g., a single blocked tube, endometriosis), it would be logical to assume that one of these problems has been preventing her from conceiving. But if the same woman's eggs fail to fertilize during a diagnostic IVF cycle, it is clear that those problems were not actually the only ones keeping her from becoming pregnant, but were "red herrings." The underlying problem preventing fertilization and conception might have gone undetected had it not been for the diagnostic ability of IVF.

The Success-Oriented Treatment Decision

Here are a few examples of how a success-oriented physician might use the information provided by these tests to determine the best course of treatment for the couple:

Blocked Fallopian tubes
If the HSG showed that one or both of the woman's tubes were blocked, the doctor would probably decide to bypass the tubes altogether and proceed directly to IVF. Theoretically,

surgery could be performed to remove the blockages. However, undetectable and untreatable damage could still remain to prevent the couple from conceiving naturally. Therefore, the doctor would probably elect not to perform a laparoscopy or any other surgical procedure to attempt to open the tubes, but instead bypass them altogether.

Highly positive anti-chlamydia antibody tests/ Normal HSG

If the HSG showed the woman's tubes to be open, but she was still unable to conceive, the doctor would probably assume that the tubal linings had been damaged—especially if the blood tests for anti-chlamydia antibodies were strongly positive. In this case, the doctor would probably elect to bypass the tubes altogether and proceed directly to IVF.

Consistently high FSH levels

If a woman's day 2 to 3 FSH was consistently as high as 20 to 25 mlU/mL (or even 15 mlU/mL), her prognosis for pregnancy with her own eggs would be considered poor. The doctor might counsel the couple to consider using donor eggs if they still wanted to try for a pregnancy.

Failure to ovulate

If a series of sonograms showed that a woman was unable to develop and/or release eggs on her own, the doctor would probably elect to try a maximum of three cycles of treatment with fertility drugs to help her ovulate and to increase her chances of conception by producing multiple eggs. Ovarian stimulation would be combined with intrauterine or intraperitoneal insemination to increase the chances of her partner's sperm meeting up with an egg. If the couple failed to conceive after 3 to 4 cycles, the doctor might advise proceeding directly to a diagnostic IVF cycle, since 85 percent of all conceptions occur within the first three treatment cycles.

Poor post-coital test

If the results of the PCT were poor, the couple would probably be advised to try intrauterine or intraperitoneal insemination to bypass the cervical mucus—probably combining IUI or IPI with fertility drugs to increase the chances of conception. If 3 to 4 cycles of this treatment failed to produce a pregnancy, the doctor would probably advise the couple to proceed to a diagnostic/therapeutic IVF cycle.

Good post-coital test/failure to conceive

If a patient who has been unable to conceive has excellent PCT results, insemination probably won't help her become pregnant. These patients should proceed directly to IVF.

Low sperm velocity/no conception with fertility drugs and insemination

The doctor would assume that the sperm is unable to fertilize the egg and would counsel the couple to proceed directly to IVF with ICSI.

An IVF cycle with no fertilization

During a standard IVF cycle, if a couple with normal-looking eggs and sperm did not achieve fertilization during the first 24 hours after retrieval, the embryologist might attempt to inject the sperm directly into the eggs (ICSI) on the second day. If this succeeded in causing fertilization, the cycle could be salvaged, although pregnancy rates are lower with second-day

ICSI. In this case, it would be difficult to know whether the initial fertilization failure was due to a problem with the egg or the sperm. If fertilization failed to occur after the second-day ICSI, during the couple's next IVF cycle, the couple might elect to fertilize 50 percent of the eggs with the partner's sperm via ICSI and leave the remaining eggs to be fertilized in the normal manner using donor sperm. The results would be interpreted as follows:

FERTILIZATION OUTCOME

DONOR SPERM	PARTNER'S SPERM/ICSI	IMPLICATION
No	No	Egg problem: consider donor eggs.
Yes	Yes	Partner's sperm had egg binding problem.
Yes	No	Probable genetic problem with partner's sperm.

Diagnostic Tests That Have Been Eliminated From the Streamlined Workup

Physical exam

Rarely, if ever, will any significant abnormality affecting reproduction and/or delivery be detected during a physical exam. If the woman has had a normal gynecological exam and pap smear within the previous 12 months, a pelvic sonogram is the only physical examination she really needs.

Cultures

It has been standard for doctors to take cervical cultures to check for infection by relevant organisms such as chlamydia. But the presence of infection with any organism other than chlamydia or gonorrhea has never been proven to cause infertility. Therefore, an extensive bacteriologic evaluation of a couple, plus prolonged, "heavy duty" antibiotic therapy, is not only not indicated but may also be potentially dangerous. Besides, a negative culture indicates only that the patient is suffering no current infection. A previous infection with chlamydia or gonorrhea could have affected her ability to conceive by damaging the Fallopian tubes. And since these organisms may not cause noticeable symptoms (or if there were symptoms, the patient may have attributed them to another cause), simply asking the woman if she has ever had a pelvic infection won't always provide accurate information. The only way to accurately assess whether or not the patient has experienced a previous pelvic infection that may have affected her fertility is via a blood test for the anti-chlamydia antibody.

Ovulation tests

In the past, a physician may have tried to assess whether a fertility patient was ovulating by asking her to keep monthly charts of her basal (first-thing-in-the-morning) body temperature (BBT) to see if it showed the mid-cycle rise that normally follows ovulation. Or the doctor may have asked her to perform a series of at-home ovulation tests or measured the level of progesterone in her blood during the latter part of her cycle to see if it showed the elevation that typically follows ovulation. Unfortunately, none of these tests are very precise. The BBT in particular is time consuming, frustrating, and can only document ovulation after it has occurred. Today we know that the most effective and efficient way to document ovulation is to actually view the egg follicle directly via a vaginal sonogram.

Endometrial biopsy

Endometrial biopsy (examination of the lining of the uterus) has traditionally been performed as a means of diagnosing luteal phase defects (insufficient progesterone production during the second half of the menstrual cycle) and evaluating the ability of the patient's uterine lining to support an implanted embryo.

Many physicians have now abandoned the endometrial biopsy, since vaginal ultrasound has provided physicians with a more sophisticated and less invasive means of evaluating the growth patterns of the patient's endometrium.

Laparoscopy

Diagnostic laparoscopy (a surgical procedure which allows the doctor to actually look inside the woman's abdominal cavity to view her pelvic organs) was once a standard component of any infertility evaluation. Laparoscopy is performed while the patient is under general anesthesia. The doctor makes several small incisions in the woman's abdomen and inflates the cavity with a small amount of carbon dioxide gas to make her organs more easily visible. A small camera, attached to a telescope, is inserted through one of the incisions. This allows the doctor to view the woman's internal anatomy on a nearby video screen. The other incisions provide access for the doctor's instruments and surgical tools.

Doctors would generally perform a laparoscopy to see if there were any signs of scar tissue or endometriosis in the woman's pelvic area, in addition to confirming tubal blockages that had been diagnosed via HSG. If any adhesions or signs of endometriosis were found, they could actually be resolved during this diagnostic procedure. If the woman failed to conceive after the laparoscopy, a second might be performed to see if the blockages or adhesions had re-occurred. Whether this type of surgery is justified as a diagnostic and treatment tool for infertility has never really been proven. For one thing, an estimated 95 percent of laparoscopies performed for diagnostic purposes reveal nothing to be wrong. Second, even if a problem is detected, there is no proof that correcting it will increase the patient's chances for conceiving. Although endometriosis seems to be associated with fertility problems, it has never been established as a *cause* of infertility. Women with endometriosis who are treated with fertility drugs and insemination have been shown to become pregnant just as often as women treated with surgery and drugs. In fact, no medical or surgical treatment of endometriosis has been shown to substantially increase fertility rates.

Anti-sperm Antibody Tests

There has been no definitive evidence that the presence of antisperm antibodies (detected via blood tests or when they are found coating the heads of the spermatozoa) causes infertility or that the success rates of either intrauterine insemination or IVF are lower in women with antisperm antibodies. In fact, 15 percent of the population who have had successful pregnancies test positive for antisperm antibodies.

Hamster Egg Penetration Test

A "high tech" test of male fertility has been the Hamster Egg Penetration Test. This test requires hamster eggs to be stripped of their outer shells (zona pellucida) and exposed to a human sperm sample. The number of sperm that penetrate the hamster egg has been considered a measure of the male's fertility.

Clinical experience has shown the hamster test to be highly unreliable. For one thing, in humans, sperm need to bind onto and penetrate the egg's outer shell (zona pellucida). This ability can't be tested in the hamster test since hamster eggs need to be stripped of their shells in order for human sperm to gain entry. Furthermore, experience has shown that a significant percentage of men who are unable to fertilize hamster eggs will actually be able to fertilize their wives eggs *in vitro,* either with or without ICSI.

SUMMARY

Since success-oriented physicians believe that most of the problems that cause infertility are impossible to diagnose and treat, the success-oriented work-up will usually consist of only a few basic, non-invasive tests to rule out obvious causes for your infertility. The workup will also help the doctor determine which form of treatment would make the best starting point for you and your partner.

The fact that success-oriented physicians believe in using IVF early on as both a diagnostic and treatment tool can save you significant time, pain, and expense in resolving your infertility.

CHAPTER 5

STEP 2:

Oral Fertility Drugs plus Intrauterine Insemination (IUI)

T he next step in The Pregnancy Prescription is a combination treatment of the oral fertility drug, clomiphene citrate (brand names: Clomid, Serophene), and intrauterine insemination (IUI). Although either treatment alone might help some couples, experience has shown that you will be more likely to conceive if the fertility drug and insemination are combined.

This step may be a good starting point for you and your partner if the results of your streamlined workup suggest any of the following:

For her:

- irregular menstrual cycles, possible lack of ovulation
- medical history suggests mild endometriosis

For him:

- a slightly low sperm count (10 to 20 million)
- somewhat decreased sperm velocity (speed of <30 microns per second) prior to processing
- an increased number of sperm with abnormal morphology (shapes)
- poor post-coital test

For both:

- unexplained infertility of more than one year duration

CLOMIPHENE CITRATE

Clomiphene citrate (Clomid, Serophene) is an oral fertility drug that initiates a process called Controlled Ovarian Hyperstimulation (COH), or superovulation, in women with normal ovulation. In COH with clomiphene citrate, the drug stimulates the hypothalamus—the control system in the brain—to produce GNRF (Gonadotropin Releasing Factor) which, in turn, causes the pituitary gland to produce additional FSH and LH. These hormones stimulate the ovary to produce greater numbers of more mature oocytes. In this way, clomiphene citrate encourages conception by helping the woman to produce additional "targets" for her mate's sperm.

How It Evolved

Clomiphene citrate was the first fertility drug to become available in this country. Ironically, clomiphene was first tested for use as a birth control pill in the 1960s. When women taking the drug were found to have an exceptionally high rate of conception, researchers decided that the best use of clomiphene would be as a means of enhancing, rather than preventing, pregnancy.

Clomiphene was originally used to treat infertile women in whom the pituitary gland and/or hypothalamus were completely unable to stimulate the production of FSH and LH, making it impossible for them to either ovulate or menstruate. Eventually, doctors started prescribing clomiphene to help increase the number of follicles produced by women who *did* ovulate normally, to increase their chances for conception.

Clomiphene Citrate as Treatment

Today, the normally prescribed dosage of clomiphene is 100 mg (two 50 mg tablets) per day for 5 to7 days, beginning on day 2 or 3 of the woman's menstrual cycle. In most cases, doses higher than 100 to 150 mg will not increase the number of follicles. Women who weigh more than 200 lbs may need more than the standard dose, and very thin women may need to take only 50 mg per day.

Clomiphene Citrate for Diagnostic Testing

Clomiphene can also be used to predict a woman's potential for becoming pregnant. For this purpose, she would take two clomiphene tablets per day starting on day 2 to 3 of her cycle, after which her ovaries would be examined via vaginal ultrasound. If the sonogram showed that she was able to produce as many as 3 to 6 mature egg follicles, it would mean that she was very responsive to the drug and would probably have a good chance of becoming pregnant. If she were to produce only one follicle, it would indicate that her ability to produce eggs was possibly compromised and her chances for pregnancy could be reduced, regardless of her chronological age.

Another test, the "clomiphene challenge test," calls for the woman to take two clomiphene tablets on days 5 to 9 of her cycle and then have her FSH level tested on day 10. If the blood test showed her FSH to be 26 or greater (the normal response would be ≤ 15) her potential for becoming pregnant would be minimal.

Women who fare poorly on either of these tests will probably not respond well to even the more potent forms of ovarian stimulation, the gonadotropins, and may need to consider other options for expanding their families.

Pros and Cons of Clomiphene Citrate

Clomiphene is a relatively inexpensive drug with limited side effects. The drug usually avoids over-stimulating (hyperstimulating) the ovaries, thus making it an extremely safe treatment option. No causal link has ever been proven between fertility drugs and ovarian or breast cancer; however, one study did note a higher incidence of ovarian cancer in women who took clomiphene citrate for more than 12 months. Since clomiphene, if it will work, will produce a pregnancy in 3 to 4 cycles, our recommendation is that women not use the drug for more than four months.

On the days clomiphene is taken, patients may experience hot flushes, mood swings, headaches, or slight visual disturbances. There is a small risk that clomiphene will have a drying effect on the cervical and endometrial mucus or cause the uterine lining to thin to the extent that it could prevent an embryo from implanting. These problems can be diagnosed via a post-coital test and/or ultrasound at the time of insemination. If the cervical mucus appears to have been adversely affected by the clomiphene, it is possible that the mucus lining the uterus and Fallopian tubes has also been negatively affected. This could interfere with the ability of the sperm or a fertilized egg to travel through the Fallopian tubes. Since these effects are completely reversed during subsequent "non-clomiphene" cycles, women experiencing these effects can plan to use other fertility drugs in subsequent cycles.

In some patients, the problem can be avoided by using a drug with a similar molecular structure as clomiphene citrate. Nolvadex™ (tamoxifen citrate), best known as an anti-breast cancer drug, works the same way as clomiphene, but without causing the drying effect in the mucus. Tamoxifen is available in 10 mg tablets, and the usual dosage is 30 to 40 mg for five days, starting on cycle day 2 or 3. When tamoxifen is substituted for clomiphene, pharmacists are often confused by the use of this drug for fertility treatment. Although it is not recognized as an ovulation-inducing agent by the FDA, tamoxifen has been found to work quite well for this purpose and costs quite a bit less than clomiphene.

INTRAUTERINE INSEMINATION (IUI)

In Intrauterine Insemination (IUI), processed semen is placed into the woman's uterus around the time that she ovulates. IUI helps to increase the chances for conception two ways. First, the pre-insemination processing helps to increase the concentration and velocity (speed) of the sperm while weeding out potential "underachievers." The insemination process itself makes it possible for the processed sperm to be deposited much closer to the oocyte than normal intercourse would permit, bypassing any potential problems in the vagina and/or cervix.

How It Evolved

IUI with processed sperm was the first effective laboratory treatment for male infertility. The first recorded inseminations were in the 1790s, when the male's ejaculate would be mechanically deposited in the vagina. From that time until the 1950s, all inseminations were carried out intravaginally, with the same "turkey baster" technique. From the 1950s through the 1970's, intravaginal insemination was replaced by intracervical insemination, in which an unprocessed ejaculate was placed into the woman's cervix so that it could mix with her cervical mucus. In the early 1980s, doctors discovered that adding tissue culture media (a nutrient broth used to grow and maintain living cells in a laboratory setting) to the semen would increase the speed with which the sperm could swim. This was found to be a way for men with low sperm counts or poor motility to increase their chances for impregnating their partners. To further enhance the chances for conception, doctors began inserting the processed sperm into the woman's uterus, bypassing the vagina and cervix completely.

Producing The Specimen

Around the time that the woman is ovulating, the male produces a sperm specimen by ejaculating into a small, sterile container. This can be done either at the doctor's office or at home. Since normal latex condoms will damage sperm, the sample should be produced through masturbation rather than via intercourse with a condom. The doctor can provide special non-latex condoms to men with religious or personal aversions to masturbation, but this method is likely to result in a good portion of the specimen being lost.

If the specimen is produced at home, it is important to keep it at room temperature until it gets to the lab, avoiding any extremes of hot or cold. In winter, one trick for keeping the sample warm is for the woman to place the closed container inside her bra, enabling her natural body heat to protect it.

The specimen should arrive at the doctor's office within two hours after it has been produced. After that time, it may begin to deteriorate...but there is no need to run red lights to get to the doctor's office to beat the deadline! Each and every sperm will not self-destruct at exactly 120 minutes after ejaculation. And even after deterioration has begun, some "resurrection" will occur during the normal processing and incubation that is a part of the standard pre-IUI preparation.

Processing the Semen

Once the sperm specimen arrives at the office, it can be processed via a number of techniques. The specific processing technique used is not critical as long as the culture media is fresh, the acid/base balance is appropriately adjusted (any deviation will kill the sperm or limit their motility), the sperm are incubated in a warm environment, and the sample is spun (placed in a centrifuge to concentrate the sperm) at the proper speed.

The sperm must be "washed" to remove the seminal plasma prior to the insemination—otherwise, the woman may suffer a mild inflammatory reaction which could cause cramping, diarrhea, or even fever. These reactions result from substances called prostaglandins, which are contained in unwashed semen. Bacteria and other cellular elements are also removed during the washing process, and antibiotics are added to the media to eliminate any remaining bacteria.

The Procedure

After the processing, which takes between 45 minutes and 2 hours, the insemination is relatively easy. The woman lies on an examining table in the usual position for a gynecological exam, and a speculum is inserted into her vagina so that the doctor can access her cervix. The doctor draws the sperm specimen up into soft plastic tubing with a syringe and then passes the tubing through the cervical opening. The woman may experience one slight cramp as the catheter passes through the cervix, and another when the catheter reaches the top of her uterus.

If the doctor has difficulty inserting the catheter, he or she may use abdominal ultrasound to help guide its placement. Once the catheter is in place, approximately 1 to 4 cc. of processed sperm is released into the uterus.

An experimental procedure called intratubal insemination, in which the sperm is placed directly into the Fallopian tubes has been suggested. In reality, this process has proven to be of little use, since it is significantly more painful, expensive, and technically more difficult than standard IUI. Besides, ultrasound studies have proven that processed sperm is perfectly able to reach the middle portion of the tube through the standard IUI technique.

A very few women may experience pain or cramping 1 to 2 hours after the insemination. This is due to a reaction to the protein in the sperm. Taking Motrin™ or another similar drug, or using a heating pad, will help relieve the cramps. Although it happens very rarely, IUI could potentially cause an infection in the woman's uterus or tubes. If she experiences chills, low abdominal pain, or an oral temperature greater than 101°F within 12 to 24 hours of the insemination, she should contact her doctor. Antibiotics administered on a timely basis can prevent permanent damage from occurring.

Exact Timing is Not Necessary

IUI needs to take place when the woman is most likely to be ovulating, but there is no need for the couple to drive themselves crazy by trying to time the insemination for the exact moment the egg is "dropped." There is actually a rather wide time frame during which fertilization can take place.

Most women will begin using a home urine test for predicting ovulation on day 12 of the cycle (women with shorter cycles lasting 25 to 26 days should start on day 10). When the results of the test are positive (meaning the LH surge has occurred and egg release can be expected within 32 to 44 hours), the woman can go ahead and schedule an ultrasound exam and the insemination for the next day, if possible.

It is very important to be examined via ultrasound prior to the insemination, since urine tests that predict ovulation can be misleading, difficult to read, or incorrect. For instance, the urine test could show a positive result on day 12 of a woman's cycle, but her ultrasound exam might show her follicles to be only 15 mm in size. This would mean that the urine test has given a false positive, which occasionally occurs in patients who have been treated with clomiphene. Since follicles grow approximately 2 mm per day, and since the target size for maturity is 20 mm, the doctor could predict that the insemination should take place 4 days later.

The timing of the actual insemination procedure is important, but not critical. Since the best time for fertilization is 36 to 48 hours after the LH surge, insemination should ideally take place during the day following the positive urine test—provided the ultrasound confirms that the test did not produce a false positive. But since pregnancy can result from exposure to sperm any time from 4 days prior to the actual ovulation to 18 hours afterwards, if the LH surge occurs on a Saturday evening and the doctor's office is closed on Sunday, Monday morning will not be too late for the insemination. Waiting any longer than 54 hours after the LH surge is risky, since the eggs will start to deteriorate and the cervical mucus will dry up beginning at around 18 hours after their release.

SUCCESS RATES

The combination of IUI and clomiphene citrate should be successful within three treatment cycles. Almost 85 percent of all pregnancies that occur with this treatment will take place during the first 6 months; 65 percent of those pregnancies will take place during the first three cycles. Repeated treatments beyond 3 cycles will be wasteful, unproductive, and frustrating. Thus, if you and your partner don't achieve a pregnancy after 3 months of clomiphene plus IUI, you should be prepared to move ahead to the next level of treatment.

Clomiphene Citrate + IUI: Donna and Frank

Donna (37-years-old) and Frank (40-years-old) had a four-year-old son who had been conceived naturally after only four months of "trying." On their son's second birthday, the couple decided it was time to give him a sibling. Since the first conception had been so easy, they didn't expect any problems. But when Donna still hadn't become pregnant after almost 2 years of well-timed intercourse, they decided to seek medical help.

Donna's evaluation was normal, and she had a low FSH (10). Frank was found to have a high sperm count, but the motility before processing was somewhat lower-than-normal.

During their first cycle of clomiphene plus IUI, Donna was given clomiphene, 100 mg per day on days 2 to 7 of her cycle. She produced only two follicles, and did not conceive. To improve her response, the doctor increased Donna's clomiphene to 150 mg/day for 7 days, but for this cycle she produced only one, single follicle. A sonogram showed her endometrium to be thin and her cervical mucus to be scant, due to the effects of the medication. Not surprisingly, the IUI was again unsuccessful.

The doctor diagnosed Donna's problem as one of egg depletion—even though she was not yet premenopausal. Her remaining oocytes were resistant to stimulation, and therefore, the doctor suspected that they would prove to be of poor genetic quality. The fact that Donna had responded poorly to the clomiphene indicated that she would not respond well to high doses of more potent fertility drugs, and that her chances for conception with her own eggs was poor.

According to their physician, continuing on to the next level of infertility treatment would not help this couple achieve a pregnancy. Donna and Frank were presented with three options:

1. They could continue trying to conceive on their own in the hope that Donna still had "a few good eggs,"one of which would develop.

2. The could try to conceive with IVF via donor eggs.

3. They could adopt.

In this couple's situation, they would have a better chance of conceiving through natural means than via IVF. Although Donna and Frank were understandably heartbroken, the success-oriented approach saved the couple years of expense and disappointment.

SUMMARY

If you have been unable to conceive due to a mild sperm problem, irregular ovulation, or unexplained infertility, the combination of clomiphene citrate plus IUI can offer you a safe, cost-effective, first step toward conception. Increasing the number of eggs and putting more sperm near them at the time of ovulation is the easiest way to enhance the natural process of conception. Approximately 20 to 30 percent of couples will conceive at this initial stage of treatment.

Clomiphene may not work for everyone, but it can give a good indication of the ovaries' ability to produce multiple follicles—a good sign, even if you don't end up conceiving by this method. If you haven't achieved a pregnancy after three cycles of this treatment, you should plan to move ahead to the next step in *The Pregnancy Prescription.*

C H A P T E R   6

STEP 3:

Injectable Fertility Drugs and Intraperitoneal Insemination (IPI)

If you have had three unsuccessful cycles with the combination of clomiphene citrate and IUI, your next step in the Pregnancy Prescription should be to maximize the potential for contact between egg and sperm through the combination of more potent fertility drugs and a procedure called intraperitoneal insemination (IPI), which allows processed sperm to be placed much closer to the newly released eggs. You will probably be a good candidate for this step if you produced multiple follicles in response to the oral medication and if your tubes appear to be open.

Although you may be tempted to proceed directly to *In vitro* fertilization (IVF) at this point, IPI is a less expensive, minimally invasive technique that deserves a try—that is, unless some additional problem has surfaced which can only be overcome via IVF.

GONADOTROPINS: THE "HEAVY HITTERS" OF FERTILITY DRUGS

The class of drugs known as gonadotropins are injectable fertility drugs that induce the woman to produce an even greater number of follicles than clomiphene citrate. Where clomiphene stimulates the hypothalamus and affects the ovary only indirectly, gonadotropins act *directly on* the ovaries to provide as many potential targets for the sperm as possible.

Which One To Choose?

The currently available gonadotropins are Pergonal, Humegon, Fertinex, and the new, genetically engineered forms of FSH: Follistim and Gonal F. Each produces comparable results, but there are differences between them. The physician will typically decide which one to use based on the makeup of the drug and its route of administration.

	MAKEUP	HOW ADMINISTERED
Pergonal	FSH+LH	Intramuscular Injection
Humegon	FSH+LH	Intramuscular Injection
Fertinex	FSH	Subcutaneous Injection
Follistim	FSH	Subcutaneous Injection
Gonal F	FSH	Subcutaneous Injection

LH has not been proven necessary for the initial stages of egg development, and theoretically, may even be detrimental. Therefore, on the basis of drug makeup, Fertinex or another pure FSH preparation may be the best choice for most women.

All of the gonadotropins need to be administered via injection, but Pergonal and Humegon must be injected intramuscularly. This means that the patient (or her partner) needs to inject the medication into the rear of the hip, near the upper buttock. The technique isn't hard to learn, but the long needle can look a bit frightening, the injection can be uncomfortable, and the idea of injecting oneself in the buttock may be hard to get used to.

Since Fertinex and the new, recombinant preparations are created from ultra-purified forms of FSH, these drugs can be administered subcutaneously. The benefit of subcutaneous injection is that it calls for a very fine needle, which allows for a greater number of easily accessible injection sites (the inner thigh, abdomen, arm, etc.). Perhaps most important though, is that the shot itself is far less painful.

Although it has been used extensively in Europe, Fertinex and the new FSH preparations are relatively new options for American doctors. Once physicians here develop a base of experience with these newer, subcutaneous forms of FSH, patient preference will probably cause them to become the drugs of choice for oocyte stimulation.

Another form of FSH, Metrodin, is currently out of production, although it had been widely used for ovarian hyperstimulation for many years. Metrodin differed from Fertinex and the newer preparations in that it needed to be administered via intramuscular—rather than subcutaneous—injection. We have no current information as to whether there are plans to reintroduce Metrodin at some future time.

Therapy with any of the gonadotropins is currently a costly undertaking. In the United States, a single ampule of

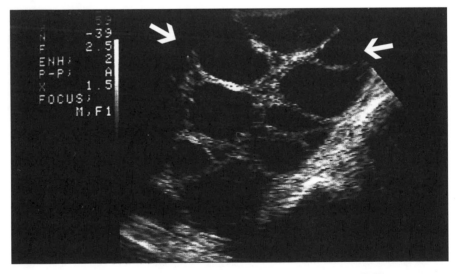

Fig. 12. *A sonographic picture of an ovary successfully stimulated with gonadotropin therapy. Note that there are at least 10 follicles present. Compare to the single ovarian follicle in Figure 1 on page 7.*

gonadotropin costs approximately $50, and patients may need to take as many as four or more ampules per day.

How Gonadotropins Are Used

Pergonal, Humegon, and Fertinex are all approximately equivalent in strength. Since patient response to these drugs is fairly predictable, daily monitoring should not be necessary—especially before the fourth or fifth day of drug administration. A typical cycle might proceed as follows:

CYCLE DAY	GONADOTROPIN DOSAGE	MONITORING
2-3	2-3 ampules/day	
4	2-3 ampules/day	
5	2-3 ampules/day	
6	2-3 ampules/day	
7	adjust dosage	blood tests, sonogram
8	adjusted dosage	
9	adjusted dosage	
10	readjusted dosage	blood tests, sonogram
11	readjusted dosage	blood tests, sonogram

When the woman's follicles have reached 20 mm in size and her estrogen level has risen to approximately 1,000 to 2,000 units, depending on how many follicles have developed, the remainder of the cycle would look like this:

CYCLE DAY	MEDICATION	PROCEDURE
12	10,000 IU of HCG at 4 to 6:00 P.M.	
13		
14		IPI

HCG causes the final stages of egg maturation to occur, and the patient should be ready for her procedure 36 to 48 hours later.

The drug Lupron, which is almost always used in an IVF cycle to help ensure that the woman's eggs will mature at approximately the same time, is not usually used in an IPI cycle. This is because IPI generally requires lower doses of gonadotropins than IVF. Eliminating Lupron also reduces the cost of an IPI cycle.

FOLLICULAR PUNCTURE/IPI

On the day of the IPI, if a sonogram shows that the follicles have already released, the doctor can proceed directly to the insemination. If it appears that the release has not yet taken place, a follicle puncture would need to be performed.

In follicular puncture, the doctor aspirates the woman's mature eggs directly from her ovaries and deposits them in the area behind the uterus (the cul de sac or Pouch of Douglas) where they would normally accumulate after ovulation. Then, with the needle still in place, the doctor injects her partner's processed sperm into the same space. This places egg and sperm in as close proximity as possible, hopefully enhancing the chances for fertilization.

How It Evolved

In the early 1980s, observations of numerous treatment cycles performed at Advanced Fertility Services showed that up to 75 percent of women who failed to conceive despite the apparently successful use of fertility drugs were actually not releasing the eggs that they had produced. Even though these women showed all the normal signs of ovulation (e.g., rise in basal body temperature, increased progesterone levels, the expected post-ovulatory changes in the uterine lining), ultrasound exams indicated that their follicles had not burst and that their eggs had not been released from the ovaries. Clearly, if an egg doesn't leave the ovary it can never make contact with the sperm or become fertilized. The retention of eggs in unruptured follicles is called the Luteinized Unruptured Follicle (LUF) Syndrome. The LUF Syndrome occurs only in 5% of natural ovulations, but much more frequently in cycles during which fertility drugs are used—even if HCG is given.

The documentation of the LUF Syndrome increased awareness of the importance of examining fertility patients via ultrasound to verify that eggs were truly being released. If the sonogram showed that the woman's follicles had not ruptured at the appropriate time, the only available remedy was for the doctor to perform a bimanual pelvic exam and actually squeeze the woman's ovary until the follicles burst. Although this technique was often effective in causing the eggs to release, it was also quite uncomfortable. One patient who had undergone the procedure said she imagined that was what it must feel like for a man to be kicked in the testicles!

By 1988, manual release was replaced by a technique called transvaginal follicle puncture, which is the same as an IVF oocyte retrieval. During this procedure, while guided by vaginal ultrasound, the doctor passes a needle through the wall of the vagina and into the ovary to draw out the mature eggs. The needle is then withdrawn from the ovary, and the doctor releases the follicular fluid, which contains the oocytes, into the Pouch of Douglas.

Once transvaginal follicle puncture was adopted, it seemed natural to take the process one step further and use an ultrasound-guided needle to place processed sperm in the Pouch of Douglas, in close proximity to the newly released eggs. This part of the procedure, intraperitoneal insemination (IPI), eliminated the need for sperm to travel through the woman's uterus and Fallopian tubes.

The combination of follicular puncture and IPI has been successful in helping a significant number of women to become pregnant and, for many couples, has eliminated the need for more invasive and expensive approaches.

The Procedure

Since the injections required for follicular puncture and IPI can be somewhat painful, the patient is usually given an intramuscular injection of Demerol (50 mg.) before it begins—even though the procedure itself is quite brief. She dons an exam gown, lies down on the table, and assumes the position for a normal gynecological exam. The sonographer inserts an ultrasound probe into her vagina to guide the doctor as the needle is inserted into the patient's ovary. Usually, all the mature follicles can be aspirated with only one needle-stick per ovary. After all the follicles have been aspirated from the ovaries, the doctor withdraws the needle without removing it from the peritoneal cavity and deposits the follicular fluid (which contains the mature oocytes) into the cul-de-sac. Then with the needle still in place, the processed sperm is deposited into the same spot, and tissue culture media is passed through the syringe to make sure that no errant eggs or sperm remain in the needle. The needle is then withdrawn from the wall of the vagina.

The combined procedure (follicular puncture + IPI) should take no more than 5 minutes and, with the use of Demerol, should not be overly painful.

Possible Implications

The fact that follicular puncture + IPI has been successful suggests that the medical community's initial assumptions regarding conception may not have been totally correct. Animal specimens and post-mortem studies have led to the traditional assumption that human fertilization takes place in the Fallopian tube. But since the removal of the oocyte from the ovary via follicular puncture combined with direct insemination of sperm into the cul-de-sac successfully causes conception, it may be true that natural fertilization takes place outside the tube, also. Perhaps sperm that are deposited in the vagina via normal intercourse make their way through the uterus and then out the ends of the Fallopian tubes, and that it is only *after the egg has been fertilized* that it is swept up by the fimbriated ends of the tube to begin its journey toward the uterus.

We believe that the cul-de-sac can be considered analogous to the petri dish in which we fertilize eggs during IVF. In IVF, we place the egg and some culture media (fluid) in a petri dish, and then add the sperm. If fertilization occurs, the embryologist draws up the embryo and places it in the woman's uterus. In nature, the egg is released into the cul-de-sac along with a good amount of follicular fluid (nature's culture media). The sperm is then added through the Fallopian tube. After fertilization, the embryo is drawn up by the fimbriated end of the tube, much as the embryologist does *In vitro*.

Safety

IPI does not appear to increase the risks associated with natural conception. There have been no reported cases of abdominal implantation of embryos created via IPI, although theoretically, this would be possible since fertilization takes place inside the body but outside the Fallopian tube. It could possibly happen that IPI would result in an increased incidence of ovarian pregnancies (the embryo could implant on the surface of the ovary) but again, this has not been reported—although it has been reported with natural conception. And although some physicians have expressed concern that IPI could lead to a higher-than-normal incidence of tubal pregnancies, more than ten years of experience with IPI has shown this fear to be unfounded.

The potential risk for Ovarian Hyperstimulation Syndrome (OHSS) with the use of gonadotropins is discussed in Chapter 7.

SUCCESS RATES

As long as the woman has at least one open (patent) tube, approximately 20 percent of couples will succeed within three cycles of gonadotropins combined with follicular puncture and IPI. If you do not achieve a pregnancy after a maximum of three cycles, you should move on to IVF, the next step in the Pregnancy Prescription.

Of the couples who go on to IVF after failing to conceive with IPI, 35 to 75 percent can be expected to become pregnant after several IVF cycles. Many of these couples will turn out to have fertilization problems that could only have been detected via IVF.

Gonadotropins + IPI: Fran and Larry

Fran (33-years-old), a secretary, and Larry (35-years-old), a teacher, had been trying to conceive for three years. Fran's evaluation showed no obvious reason for her failure to become pregnant. Her blood test for antichlamydia antibodies was negative, and her tubes appeared to be open. Ultrasound exams showed her to be ovulating.

Because her husband's semen analysis showed that Larry had a "borderline" specimen, with sperm that was classified as "subnormal" with respect to shape and motility, the doctor decided to help nature along with a trial of clomiphene citrate and IUI. Fran responded well to the medication and produced 4 to 6 follicles during each of three cycles but, the couple still didn't conceive.

Since nature obviously needed even more of a helping hand, the doctor offered the couple a choice between IPI and IVF for their next cycle. But their savings account was becoming rapidly depleted, and they elected to try one cycle of the less costly option—IPI—before moving ahead to IVF.

Fran was instructed to take 4 ampules of Fertinex on days 2 and 3 of her next cycle, and then 2 amps per day until day 10. When Fran saw the doctor for monitoring on day 11, he discovered that she had produced 10 mature follicles. He had her take HCG that evening, and a follicle puncture/IPI was performed on day 13. The doctor aspirated 6 follicles from her right ovary and injected

Larry's processed sperm into her cul de sac. Four weeks later, an ultrasound showed a gestational sac in Fran's uterus, and the couple was delighted to learn that at last, she was pregnant.

SUMMARY

The injectable fertility drugs known as gonadotropins can help a woman produce greater numbers of mature eggs than clomiphene citrate. Combining gonadotropin therapy with follicular puncture and intraperitoneal insemination can help ensure that multiple oocytes will be released from the ovary and that freshly processed sperm will end up in close proximity to these newly released eggs.

Since IPI is cost-effective and minimally invasive, this treatment is the next logical step for patients who are responsive to fertility drugs and appear to have normal tubal function. Couples who don't succeed after three cycles with gonadotropins and IPI should move ahead to the next step: *In vitro* fertilization.

STEP 4A:

In Vitro Fertilization (IVF): Oocyte Stimulation and Retrieval

If you have already gone through IUI and IPI without becoming pregnant, you are probably feeling very discouraged. But please don't lose hope. You still have a good chance of conceiving the child you want so desperately—but in your case, nature may need some extra help from modern technology.

If you have not conceived after a *maximum* of six cycles of fertility drugs combined with insemination, IVF should be your next step in the Pregnancy Prescription. Couples who have been diagnosed with any of the following may want to *begin* their fertility treatment with IVF:

- Extremely poor sperm quality: count of less than 5 million after processing; velocity (speed) less than 60 mic/second after processing; and/or very poor morphology (shape)
- Both Fallopian tubes are completely blocked
- One Fallopian tube is blocked *plus* the woman has tested positive for anti-chlamydial antibodies
- A previous history of ectopic pregnancy and failure to conceive after at least one year of unprotected intercourse
- Severe endometriosis, with or without a history of surgery
- Longstanding (3 to 4 years), unexplained infertility— particularly if the woman is in her mid-thirties

A typical IVF cycle includes the following phases:

1. Stimulation of egg follicles
2. Monitoring of follicle development
3. Oocyte retrieval
4. Fertilization
5. Embryo transfer

STIMULATION

To maximize the chances for a successful IVF cycle, the doctor will use drugs to stimulate the ovaries to produce rather large numbers of high-quality eggs that will mature at approximately the same rate. He or she will decide which medications to use and how to use them based upon the individual characteristics of each patient.

The most important drugs used during the stimulation phase of an IVF cycle are gonadotopins—e.g., Fertinex (FSH)—and Lupron (leuprolide acetate, a form of Gonadotropin Releasing Hormone—GnRH—blocking agent). The gonadotropins stimulate the ovaries to produce multiple egg follicles, and the Lupron synchronizes the development of those eggs. Whenever injectable fertility drugs are used, HCG (Human Chorionic Gonadotropin) must be taken at the proper time to bring the eggs to their final stage of maturity and prepare them for retrieval.

Fertinex (FSH)

The first injectable fertility drug ever used for IVF was Pergonal, which is made of a combination of FSH and LH. Since the early days of IVF, it has been discovered that LH is not crucial to stimulating egg development. Today, Fertinex, which contains only FSH, is the preferred drug for oocyte stimulation. We rarely use Pergonal or Humegon, which also consists of both FSH and LH.

Fertinex is relatively new to the United States, having first become available here in November, 1996. European experience showed us that Fertinex was interchangeable with Metrodin, a drug that is no longer available in this country, and that the two drugs produced equivalent results. The difference was that, since

Fertinex is highly purified, this newer drug could be injected sub-cutaneously (beneath the skin) with a very small needle, while Metrodin needed to be administered with a larger needle and via intramuscular injection. This important difference made Fertinex a far easier, more comfortable drug to use. For this reason, Fertinex is the current drug-of-choice for pre-IVF follicle stimulation.

Women who do not respond to injectable fertility drugs should probably not make more than two attempts at IVF. Even if such a woman was eventually able to produce one or more eggs, and those eggs went on to become fertilized, her chances for a pregnancy would still be low.

Lupron

Lupron suppresses the natural activity of a woman's ovaries. This makes it possible for the follicles that are generated via stimulation by Fertinex to develop more uniformally and to reach maturity at approximately the same time. Such synchronization is critical, since a woman's eggs need to be at exactly the right stage in their development when they are exposed to the sperm. Fertilization can only occur during the stage known as Metaphase II, which is the point at which the number of chromosomes contained in the egg reduces from 46 to 23. If Metaphase II has not yet occurred at the time of the IVF retrieval, the eggs will contain too much genetic material (46 chromosomes) and will either be unable to become fertilized or produce an abnormal embryo containing excess genetic material.

Since adopting Lupron for use in IVF, pregnancy rates have greatly improved. In fact, even in studies that show equivalent numbers of embryos to be produced both with and without

Lupron, there appear to be more pregnancies among the women taking Lupron.

There is another important benefit to using Lupron for IVF. When a woman is preparing for IVF, she is so focused on what's going on in her ovaries that she may worry that she will ovulate on her own before the retrieval. If that were to happen, the IVF cycle would have to be cancelled. With Lupron, it is virtually impossible for woman's follicles to release spontaneously.

With the benefits of Lupron also comes a disadvantage: women taking Lupron require higher dosages of gonadotropins. In addition, women in their late 30's may not respond well to the drug. In these patients, Lupron can impair the ability of the ovary to produce any follicles at all, even with high doses of Fertinex.

Lupron can be administered in various dosages and at various times in the menstrual cycle, depending on the patient's individual characteristics and on her unique pattern of ovarian response. The two most common dosing regimens are the "Long Lupron" and the "Flare" protocols.

Long Lupron Protocol

With this regimen, the woman begins taking her Lupron injections during the last week of the menstrual period that *precedes* her IVF cycle. The purpose of starting the injections at this time is to prevent the *following* month's eggs from beginning to be stimulated, since eggs are actually "recruited" for a particular cycle during the one that precedes it. This ensures that the only eggs developed for the IVF cycle are those stimulated via the FSH injections.

Flare Protocol

When Lupron is begun on day 2 to 3 of the woman's IVF cycle, this is called the "Flare" protocol. This regimen generally has the opposite effect of the "Long Lupron" protocol in that, given *early* in the menstrual cycle, Lupron tends to cause an outpouring of FSH and LH from the pituitary gland before it begins to suppress the production of these hormones. A variation on the Flare protocol—the "Microdose Flare"—has been found useful for women who respond poorly to stimulation.

Combining Medications for Optimal Results

To predict which medications are most likely to produce the best results, doctors evaluate each patient as to whether she is most likely to be a normal responder, low responder, or over-responder. When it comes to prescribing fertility drugs, patients in each of these groups have their own special needs.

The Normal Responder: A woman in her twenties to mid-thirties with a low FSH level on day 2 to 3 of her cycle.

BEGINNING ON DAY	MEDICATION	ACTION
21 of previous cycle	1 mg. Lupron/day	
1 of IVF cycle	reduce to .5 mg Lupron/day	
2-3 of IVF cycle	continue .5 mg Lupron/day add 4 amps Fertinex/day	
5-6 of IVF cycle	continue Lupron/ adjust dose of Fertinex	blood tests/ sonogram
9-10 of IVF cycle	continue Lupron/ adjust dose of Fertinex	blood tests/ sonogram
11 of IVF cycle	discontinue Lupron, Fertinex; take HCG at 9:00 P.M.	
9:00 A.M., day 13		EGG RETRIEVAL

Specific dosages of Lupron and Fertinex will vary, depending on how well the woman responds to the drug. The daily dosage of Fertinex may range from 2 to 10 amps per day. However, the patient who doesn't produce multiple follicles with 4 to 6 amps will rarely produce additional follicles despite an increased dose. Reducing her Lupron and increasing her Fertinex may cause such a woman to produce a greater number of egg follicles, but her chances of becoming pregnant will probably not improve.

The Low Responder: The woman with an FSH level of 10 to 15 mlU/mL on cycle day two. These women generally do better with the "Flare" protocol:

BEGINNING ON DAY	MEDICATION	ACTION
2 of IVF cycle	microdose Lupron twice daily	
5 of IVF cycle	continue Lupron and add 6 amps Fertinex	
9-10 of IVF cycle	adjust Fertinex dosage	blood tests/ sonogram
11 of IVF cycle	discontinue Lupron and Fertinex; take HCG at 9:00 P.M.	blood tests/ sonogram
13 of IVF cycle, 9:00 A.M		EGG RETRIEVAL

A second option for low responders is the "Microdose Flare," which calls for injecting 1/400 the normal Lupron dose morning and evening, starting on day 2 of the woman's cycle. She would then begin taking relatively high doses of Fertinex on day 4 to 5.

Still another dosing technique for the low responder is to begin 1 mg of Lupron on day 21 of the cycle preceding the IVF cycle and to discontinue the Lupron when the woman gets her period. She would then begin stimulation on day 2 to 3 with 6 to 8 daily ampules of Metrodin alone.

The most recent protocol is called the "Parlodel rebound" method, which has been reported by a group of Japanese physicians to enhance the stimulation of low responders. A course of Parlodel, a medication to reduce the woman's prolactin level, is taken before treatment with Fertinex is begun. The doctors speculate that using Parlodel to lower an already normal prolactin level should enhance follicle stimulation. Although this novel approach needs time to be evaluated, it might be worth trying. The addition of Parlodel would add little in the way of risk or expense, and any mild side effects (nausea, dizziness) could be managed by having the patient begin with one-half the normal dose and to take it with milk at bedtime.

The Overresponder

Overresponders are women who produce extremely high numbers of egg follicles. These follicles tend to contain many eggs, but the eggs are usually of poor quality. They do not develop normally in terms of size or maturity and result in lower pregnancy rates than would be expected.

Overresponders are the most difficult patients for the physician to manage. Since overresponders are likely to produce very high levels of estrogen with rather small follicles, these patients run the highest risk of cycle cancellation and hospitalization for Ovarian Hyperstimulation Syndrome (OHSS). In overresponders, it is very important that the natural activity of the ovaries be suppressed prior to stimulation with gonadotropins and that the egg follicles be allowed to develop very slowly. This can make a big difference in the quality of the eggs produced and in the resulting pregnancy rates.

One potential drug protocol for a woman who qualifies as an overresponder is to have her take birth control pills for 17-or-more days to put the ovaries at rest. After the birth control pills have been discontinued, the woman would begin taking a daily dose of 1 mg of Lupron, to further "shut down" her ovaries. After 7 to14 days of Lupron, she would add two daily ampules of Fertinex, and then four days later, she would visit the doctor's office for monitoring. Depending on the results of the blood tests and sonogram, her Fertinex dosage might be adjusted upward in small levels, since follicles tend to develop very quickly in these women.

Another option for the overresponder is to have her take a single injection of Depot (long-acting) Lupron on day 1 to 5 of her menstrual cycle. This would cause her ovaries to be at rest for approximately one month. Since it has been shown that over-responders produce the best quality eggs when their ovaries have been shut down for long periods, the injection would be repeated 30 days later. Several weeks after the second Depot Lupron injection, the woman could begin taking low doses of Fertinex to stimulate egg production.

Potential Risks of Controlled Ovarian Hyperstimulation

Hyperstimulation is a small but necessary risk associated with the use of gonadotropins. In fact, all women who respond well to stimulation can be said to be hyperstimulated to some extent. However, in Ovarian Hyperstimulation Syndrome (OHSS), an unidentified substance causes the fluid component of blood to seep through the walls of the blood vessels into the patient's abdomen and chest cavities. The dangerous result is that the blood becomes too concentrated (thick) and may be excessively prone to clotting.

Although all women on fertility drugs experience some degree of bloating and discomfort, these symptoms are usually more severe in patients with OHSS. Women with OHSS may also experience severe abdominal distention and shortness of breath. The symptoms do not occur until 96 hours after the HCG injection

OHSS can occur when the ovaries produce higher-than-desired estrogen levels (3000 to 4000 picograms/ml, with 1200 to 2000 being the normal target) and dramatically large numbers (e.g. 40 to 50) of developing follicles. But not all women who have high levels of estrogen and large numbers of follicles develop OHSS. The problem occurs (to some limited extent) only in about 15 to 20 percent of cycles in which injectable fertility drugs are used. Hyperstimulation rarely, if ever, occurs with clomiphene citrate.

It is usually possible to predict which patients are at high risk for developing OHSS. These women tend to develop numerous 10 to 12 mm follicles in addition to a number of normal sized, 20 mm ones, and their estrogen levels may exceed 5000 picograms/ml. The need to screen for OHSS is just one of the reasons monitoring is necessary whenever gonadotropins are used.

Hyperstimulation syndrome can be prevented if HCG is withheld for that cycle, but to do so would mean that the IVF cycle would have to be cancelled. Although the package insert for gonadotropins recommends that HCG not be administered if the patient's estrogen level exceeds 2000, most women can produce estrogen in the 2,000 to 4,000 picograms/ml range without developing problems. In clinical practice, HCG is commonly given in those circumstances.

Since hyperstimulation syndrome always resolves when a woman gets her period, the problem is self-limiting. But if the woman conceives, it can worsen dramatically—especially if she has a multiple pregnancy. Therefore, if a woman appears to be at extreme risk for OHSS, any embryos that develop can be frozen for use during a subsequent cycle. The good news is that, even if a patient does go on to develop OHSS, her risk of serious illness is low. Hospitalization is required in only about 1/800 cases, and the disorder rarely progresses to a life-threatening situation. Worldwide, only two fatalities from OHSS have been reported during the last 25 years.

There are two types of hyperstimulation: early and late.

Early Hyperstimulation
Early hyperstimulation results from the HCG injection and occurs some 96 hours after it has been given. This type of hyperstimulation occurs most often in women with polycystic ovaries (overresponders) who have developed numerous tiny follicles in addition to the ones that have developed to maturity and been retrieved. Doctors can usually predict which patients will experience this type of hyperstimulation based on whether the sonogram demonstrates that multiple small follicles are present in the ovaries.

The key to determining the potential level of seriousness for a case of hyperstimulation is to evaluate how concentrated the woman's blood has become. If too much water has migrated from the woman's blood circulatory system into her abdominal cavity, her red blood cell count will be too high (hematocrit > 50 percent; normal is 35 to 40 percent), which means that her blood is too concentrated. A mild degree of early hyperstimulation may not be cause for concern, but if the problem is moderate-to-severe, the patient will need to be hospitalized and given intravenous protein fluid to recapture liquid back into her circulatory system. In some women, it may become necessary to pass a needle through the vagina into the abdominal cavity, where it can withdraw a significant amount (1 to 2 quarts) of the excess fluid. This procedure will also help to relieve the patient's discomfort.

Late Hyperstimulation

Late hyperstimulation occurs approximately one week after the embryo transfer. In these cases, starting at about 3 to 5 days after the transfer, the woman notices that her ovaries have become distended and fluid has accumulated in her abdomen. This almost always means that the woman has conceived and that the hyperstimulation syndrome is associated with a pregnancy. Often, pregnancies associated with late hyperstimulation are multiple gestations that result in twins or triplets. Hospitalization is frequently necessary, but the problem is almost always self-limiting. Knowing they are pregnant tends to compensate these women for whatever treatment they need to endure!

MONITORING

IVF patients need to be monitored to evaluate the quality and quantity of egg follicles produced. This monitoring is performed via blood hormone testing and vaginal sonogram. The results of the blood tests and sonogram need to be evaluated together to help the doctor decide how best to proceed with a patient.

Monitoring is virtually never needed before a woman has had at least 5 to 6 days of stimulation, except in cases where the woman has polycystic ovaries. Waiting until later in the cycle to begin monitoring can help to make IVF significantly more convenient and cost-effective without compromising either patient safety or the potential success of the procedure.

Ultrasound

Vaginal ultrasound enables the doctor to evaluate the number and size of the follicles the patient is producing. Since follicle size is the single most important criteria for determining the optimal time for egg retrieval, once the majority of the developing follicles have reached 20 mm in size, HCG can be taken and the retrieval can be planned.

Blood Hormone Levels

The two hormones that need to be monitored for an IVF cycle are estrogen, which is produced by the ovaries, and progesterone, which is produced by the cells that surround the ovary.

Estrogen

A woman's blood estrogen level, which is the second most important criteria for timing the patient's retrieval, increases as the number and size of her developing egg follicles increase. Both the number *and* size of the follicles contribute to the level of estrogen development. For example, if a woman has only 5 to 6 developing follicles measuring 18 to 20 mm, and her estrogen is measured at 1200 pg/ml, that level may signal that the follicles have reached maturity and she is ready for her HCG injection. However, if that same level of estrogen were seen in a woman with many follicles measuring only 10 to12 mm each, it would mean that she was overresponding to the medication and that her dosage needed to be drastically reduced or discontinued.

Progesterone

The third most important criteria for determining a woman's readiness for retrieval is her blood progesterone level. As with estrogen, a woman's progesterone level depends on the number and size of the eggs she has produced. The initial rise in progesterone, which usually occurs with the LH surge or HCG injection, is the first sign that the lining of her uterus is being prepared for potential implantation by an embryo.

Occasionally, a woman's progesterone level will increase prematurely to a level of more than 4.0 ng/ml prior to administration of the HCG. This may mean that her uterine lining is not well-synchronized with the other elements of her cycle. In such cases, the woman can proceed with the retrieval, but her embryos should be frozen for use during a later cycle. Under certain conditions, a woman with a very high number of eggs will also have a high progesterone level despite the fact that her uterine lining appears to be of the appropriate thickness. In that situation, the fresh embryos can be transferred according to the usual procedures.

THE RETRIEVAL

The procedure to remove the mature egg follicles is probably the part of the IVF process that is most-feared by potential patients. Happily, most women who go through a retrieval today agree that it is not such a big deal.

Prior to 1986, the only way to retrieve eggs was via laparoscopy—a surgical procedure that required general anesthesia, took between one and two hours to perform, and left the woman with incisions to heal, stitches to remove, and a significant degree of discomfort for days afterward. Today, all that has changed, and egg retrieval is no longer a surgical procedure. Instead, the eggs are removed via an ultrasound-guided needle placed through the wall of the vagina and into the ovary. The procedure is extremely safe, provides minimal discomfort, and rarely takes more than 10 minutes.

Before the Retrieval

The patient should not eat solid foods after the midnight prior to the retrieval. She may, however, have a cup of coffee or tea in the morning.

It is advisable for the couple to abstain from sexual activity for the 2 days prior to the retrieval to ensure the highest possible sperm count for the male.

On Retrieval Day

Preparation

The patient will undress, put on an examining gown, and empty her bladder. She will lie down on the exam table and be positioned in the same way as for routine sonograms or gynecological exams. Then she will be hooked up to an electrocardiogram machine and have a blood pressure cuff wrapped around her arm, so that her vital signs may be monitored throughout the procedure. An IV line will be placed into her arm, and she will be put under light conscious sedation with a medication called Versed (a tranquilizer similar to Valium) along with a pain killer such as Demerol. The medications will keep the patient from experiencing any significant discomfort during the procedure and will allow her to remain conscious, albeit relaxed and drowsy.

The Procedure

During the retrieval, the sonographer, doctor, and nurse work together. The doctor inserts the needle through the wall of the vagina and into each ovary under the guidance of the vaginal ultrasound wand, and aspirates the mature follicles. Generally, all the eggs in an ovary can be recovered with a single puncture. As the follicles are aspirated, the couple can watch the video monitor and actually see them collapse as the ovaries return to a more normal size. The test tubes in which the eggs are trapped are then handed over to the embryologist in the IVF laboratory. The embryologist locates the eggs under a microscope and puts them into an incubator.

After the Retrieval

The patient usually rests for 1 to 2 hours after the retrieval, after which she is able to go home. The medications used during the procedure are extremely safe, but the patient is asked not to drive or perform any dangerous or delicate tasks for the next 24 hours because her coordination may be impaired. She may experience some mild cramps, dizziness, and/or vaginal staining after the procedure, but these have usually subsided by the time she is ready to leave the recovery area.

Although there is an extremely low complication rate from the retrieval process, any time a needle is passed into the human body there is the potential for infection or internal bleeding. Thankfully, these occur very infrequently with retrievals. During the last 8 to 10 years, only 1 to 2 fatalities *worldwide* have been attributed to egg retrieval, out of a total of some 750,000 total procedures performed.

SUMMARY

Doctors use a variety of drugs to help stimulate women to produce multiple follicles for IVF. These drugs can be used in many different combinations and at varying dosage strengths suitable to individual patient needs. Regular monitoring via ultrasound and blood hormone testing helps the doctor to continuously adjust the patient's medications for the best possible results. The retrieval itself is a relatively safe, easy, and pain-free procedure.

CHAPTER 8

STEP 4B:

In Vitro Fertilization (IVF): Fertilization and the Embryo Transfer

Eggs are a critical element in IVF—but even with the most up-to-date techniques, you still can't make a baby without sperm. Nevertheless, it is no longer necessary for the male to produce millions, thousands, or even hundreds of sperm in order for conception to take place. With today's IVF technology, pregnancy is possible even if there is just one live sperm available to unite with a single mature egg.

THE SPERM SPECIMEN

Compared to an oocyte retrieval, the man has a relatively easy time of it. He needs only to produce a sperm specimen to be used to fertilize the retrieved eggs. Some time after the retrieval, the male will be asked to ejaculate into a sterile specimen container, which he will then give directly to the embryologist and/or andrologist. (Don't worry—a private area is always provided for this step!) The sperm is "processed" and separated from the seminal fluid via one of several different techniques and then used for *In vitro* insemination.

Some men may have no sperm at all (azoospermia) in their ejaculate. This can result from blockages in the epididymal ducts that lead from the testes, having been born without such ducts, or by a direct impairment in the ability of the testicles to produce sperm. Whatever the cause, the condition usually condemned such men to a lifetime of absolute sterility. But now, there are two techniques that may be used to extract sperm directly from the testicles: Microsurgical Epididymal Sperm Aspiration (MESA) and Testicular Sperm Extraction (TESE).

Microsurgical Epididymal Sperm Aspiration (MESA)

MESA is used to extract sperm from men with obstructions in their epididymal ducts. In this microsurgical procedure, which is performed with a local anesthetic while the patient is under conscious sedation (Demerol, Versed), the physician attempts to locate an area near the end of the epididymal tubule that contains live sperm, removes as many as possible, and gives the specimen to the embryologist to prepare for ICSI. Sperm removed via this method can also be frozen for subsequent IVF cycles. MESA is performed on the same day as the egg retrieval and takes about one hour to perform.

Interestingly, it had always been believed that sperm that had not matured during the trip through the epididymis would be too immature to fertilize eggs. This has been proven untrue. In fact, sperm from the near (proximal) end have been shown to be best for fertilizing eggs, while sperm from the far (distal) end have consistently failed to achieve fertilization *In vitro* with ICSI. The near end of the epididymis is now the area of choice for retrieving sperm from men with obstructions.

Testicular Sperm Extraction (TESE)

TESE is another outpatient surgical procedure, performed on the same day as the egg retrieval while the male is under conscious sedation (and with the testes numbed via local anesthetic). For TESE, a small incision is made in the scrotum, one testicle is exposed, and several small pieces of the testicle are extracted (as in a testicular biopsy). If necessary for diagnostic purposes, a testicular biopsy can be performed at the same time. The embryologist examines the removed tissue under a microscope and selects individual sperm to inject into the eggs.

Although sperm harvested via TESE yield similar fertilization rates as MESA, the sperm from the testes are more difficult for the embryologist to work with since they exhibit very little movement. In addition, they must be separated from other testicular cells before processing. At this time, it is not possible to freeze testicular tissue; however, various techniques for doing so are being evaluated.

TESE takes less than 30 minutes to perform, and the patient will be able to go home after 2 to 3 hours and be able to return to work the next day or so. He will have sore testes for approximately one week.

For both MESA and TESE, the patient will be unable to drive a car for 24 hours after the procedure due to the effects of sedation.

MESA and TESE Success Rates

Both MESA and TESE make the successful outcome of an IVF cycle even more difficult, since another variable—obtaining viable sperm—has been added. Although sperm obtained via MESA and TESE yield good fertilization rates with ICSI (50 to 80 percent), pregnancy rates cannot be expected to be equally high. The real key to predicting the chances for a successful outcome with MESA/TESE is the age of the female partner, her ability to produce many ooctyes, and any history of previous pregnancies. If a woman is 38- to 40-years-old and produces only 3 to 4 oocytes in response to fertility drugs, chances for a successful outcome are unlikely and this treatment option is not advised. If, however, the female partner is young and produces many oocytes, pregnancy rates are similar to regular IVF.

When a testicular biopsy is necessary to evaluate azoospermia, if the female partner is a good candidate for IVF, the biopsy should be performed on the day of the egg retrieval. This will enable the doctor to harvest some sperm for ICSI and give the couple a chance for a pregnancy at the same time that the diagnostic procedure is being performed.

FERTILIZATION

The three most important elements for maximizing the chances for successful egg fertilization are: the skill of the embryologist, the caliber of the IVF lab, and the quality and maturity of the eggs.

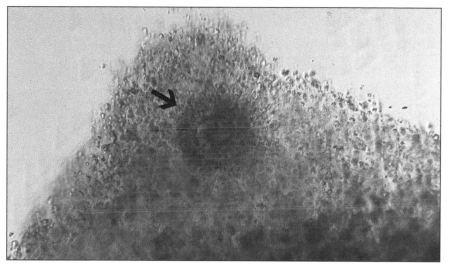

Fig. 13. *An egg in follicular fluid located by the embryologist under a microscope.*

The Embryologist

An embryologist is typically a PhD who has been trained in techniques for growing and maintaining cells in tissue culture systems in the laboratory. Since the embryologist maintains full responsibility for the IVF lab, he or she must be meticulous in adhering to high standards of technique and excellent quality control.

Among the many functions performed in the IVF lab are:

1. Locating the eggs within the follicular fluid that is removed from the ovary

2. Grading the eggs in terms of maturity

3. Maintaining media and culture conditions that will allow the cells to grow for the required period of time

4. Performing micromanipulation (ICSI, Assisted Hatching)

Since fertilization rates depend on egg quality, a critical responsibility of the embryologist is to evaluate the newly-retrieved eggs in terms of maturity and structural integrity. The embryologist can gauge the maturity of an egg by examining the crown of cells that surround it (the corona radiata). If these surrounding cells appear expanded or enlarged, and have a specific, recognizable look, the egg can be assumed to have reached Metaphase II and be ready for fertilization. If the eggs appear immature, however, the eggs will be maintained in the incubator and fertilization will be delayed until Metaphase II has been achieved.

If a couple's fertilization rates turn out to be much poorer than had been predicted, it may mean either that the eggs were less mature than could be predicted by their outward appearance, or that the eggs were just of poor quality.

It was once believed that stripping immature eggs of their surrounding cells would assist the fertilization process. We now know that this practice interferes with nature and can actually impede fertilization—except when the sperm needs to be injected directly inside the egg.

The IVF Laboratory

One of the best ways to evaluate the quality of an IVF center is through the fertilization and embryonic growth rates achieved by the lab. The quality of the IVF laboratory is generally an all-or-nothing proposition; that is, a lab that is not well-run will produce *zero* pregnancies, while a well-run lab may produce either many or few pregnancies, depending on the age of the female patients and other patient-selection criteria.

Today, the techniques, equipment, and culture media used to fertilize eggs and grow embryos are quite standardized. The majority of labs maintain their living cells in a fluid culture media that has been commercially produced using strict standards of quality control. This is a vast difference from the early days of IVF, when each lab had to produce its own media—the quality of which was easily compromised based on impurities or an unfavorable mineral content in the water that was the basis for the media. Most IVF labs today also use similar types of incubators to house their developing eggs and embryos. The only trick is that the incubators need to be carefully maintained and observed so that the carbon dioxide content and pH are well-maintained (any change in the acid/base balance can adversely affect embryonic growth). In fact, virtually all of today's embryos are cultured underneath a layer of mineral oil, which serves both to assure strict control of the media pH and to shield the embryo from impurities.

Co-culture

The concept of co-culture calls for the addition of living cells to the commercially-produced media that is normally used to maintain the eggs, sperm, and developing embryos. These cells may come from such sources as the endometrium or Fallopian tubes

113

of a cow, the woman's own endometrial cells, cells from another woman, or a specialized strain of tissue culture cells. Experts believe that the addition of these "helper cells" increases the biological "naturalness" of the environment and produces better-quality embryos.

We prefer using the patient's own granulosa cells (the cells that surround the egg when it is removed from the follicle) as co-culture cells, since this technique limits the theoretical possibility of transferring foreign viruses—whether they are produced by an animal or another human—to the embryo.

The Process of Fertilization

If the embryologist finds the retrieved eggs to be at the proper stage of maturity (Metaphase II), he/she will place several in each petri dish in the appropriate culture media. Some 25,000 to100,000 of the most active sperm will then be added to each container in hopes that one spermatozoa will be able to penetrate each egg.

If the embryologist has noticed that, after processing, the sperm are moving at too low a velocity to make natural penetration of the egg likely (in our laboratory, less than 60 microns/second), fertilization can be facilitated by the injection of a single sperm directly into each egg. This procedure is called Intracytoplasmic Sperm Injection (ICSI).

Intracytoplasmic Sperm Injection

Perhaps the most exciting scientific breakthrough to occur in reproductive medicine has been the development of ICSI. ICSI has revolutionized the process of infertility treatment by making it possible for men with even extremely poor sperm counts and barely twitching motility to fertilize their partners' eggs with

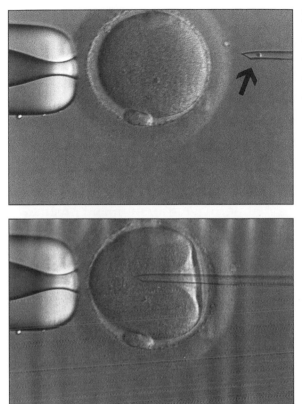

Fig. 14. *ICSI: While the egg is held in place by a microscopic suction instrument, a sperm, contained in the needle, is ready to be injected into the egg.*

Fig. 15. *ICSI-2: The sperm injection.*

approximately the same success rates (60 percent) as men with normal sperm counts.

ICSI is an extremely delicate microsurgical technique which demands great skill by the embryologist. The target—the egg—measures only 1/100 of the size of a pinhead, and the sperm is a mere 1/400 of the size of the egg.

Before ICSI can be performed, the embryologist must strip the eggs of their surrounding cells. This allows a detailed evaluation to make sure the eggs are at the proper stage of maturity. If the eggs have not yet reached Metaphase II, the procedure may need to be delayed several hours until they do so.

To perform ICSI, the embryologist places the active sperm in an immobilizing fluid medium. Then, using a very fine needle, he/she breaks the tail of the sperm to render it incapable of moving, picks it up, and injects it into the egg. If fertilization occurs, two pronuclei will become visible within 16 to 18 hours after the injection, and cell division will occur approximately 12 hours later. Interestingly, embryos created via ICSI often look more healthy than those created via natural (IVF) fertilization.

Experience has shown that normal fertilization and pregnancy rates can be achieved with ICSI even with sperm that are morphologically abnormal (irregularly-shaped). These findings challenge the long-held belief that abnormally-shaped sperm are likely to be genetically impaired and thus incapable of fertilizing an egg. They also challenge the concept that surgery is the only treatment option for a man with an abnormal sperm count thought to be related to a varicocele—a varicose vein in the testicle which is alleged to cause male infertility through the production of abnormally-shaped sperm.

Because ICSI results in such high fertilization rates, we use ICSI if we have any reason at all to suspect that a male's sperm will be incapable of fertilizing his partner's eggs. We base these suspicions on such factors as poor fertilization during a previous IVF cycle, poor post-processing velocity of the sperm specimen, or sperm that appear to be abnormally shaped. Since there is a markedly lower pregnancy rate when ICSI is performed on the second day after retrieval, we prefer to err on the side of being aggressive and perform ICSI on the day of the retrieval whenever it appears likely that the procedure will ultimately be necessary.

Assisted Hatching

In the body, after the egg has fertilized (either with or without ICSI) and the embryo has undergone numerous cell divisions and contains hundreds of cells within the zona pellucida (outer covering), the zona must break to allow the embryo room for further expansion and implantation. However, certain patients produce embryos which appear to be viable, but are unable to break out of the zona. These patients may benefit from assisted hatching. In this micromanipulation technique, the embryologist thins areas of the zona pellucida using a very dilute biological enzyme. This procedure, which thins the zona pellucida, is performed when the embryo is at the 8-cell stage or later, just before the embryo transfer.

Assisted hatching may be used in patients who have failed to achieve pregnancy despite transfers of healthy-looking embryos in previous cycles. The technique may help increase the chances for pregnancy in women in their late thirties, as well as for those whose embryos appear to have thickened zona pellucidae.

THE EMBRYO TRANSFER

Timing

Once fertilization has taken place, the embryo transfer may take place anywhere from 1 to 6 days later.

In the early years of IVF, embryo transfer was always performed after 2 days, at the 2 to 4 cell stage. The laboratory expertise had not yet been developed to allow a developing embryo to survive outside the woman's body for a longer period than that. Many embryologists now believe that 2 days was probably not sufficient to allow the lining of the uterus to become sufficiently

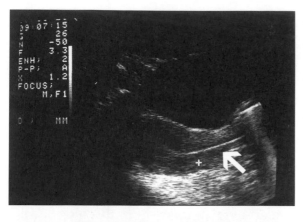

Fig. 16. *Sonigraphically guided embryo transfer. The catheter (white line on the left side) is inserted through the cervix.*

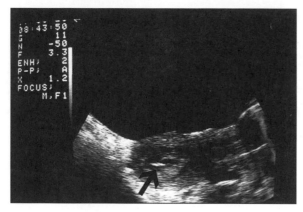

Fig. 17. *The lining of the uterus surrounds a bright white area in the center of the uterus. This is a reflection of the embryo transfer medium insuring accurate embryo transfer.*

mature for implantation, since with natural conception, it takes a newly-formed embryo 5 to 7 days to make its way through the Fallopian tubes to implant into the uterus. Theoretically, a number of potentially viable embryos may have been lost due to an immature endometrium.

Thanks to improved culture media and the use of co-culture, embryos can now be sustained outside of the uterus for a much longer period of time than was previously possible. Today, the majority of IVF centers routinely transfer embryos at 72 instead of 24 to 48 hours. In addition to allowing the uterine lining to develop more fully, this additional time gives the embryologist the opportunity to evaluate the embryos as they develop. Some eggs may fertilize initially, but then the embryo might stop dividing between the 2- and 6-cell stage. Other embryos may divide too slowly. If an embryo is incapable of reaching at least the 6-cell, if not the 8-cell stage by day 3, it is a sign that the embryo is of poor quality and would have been incapable of growing in the uterus to become a clinical pregnancy.

Another advantage to a longer observation period is that the embryos can be observed to see if they begin to fragment. This means that certain cells in the embryo, called blastomeres, break up over time. If developing embryos fragment, it usually means that there was a chromosomal abnormality in the egg, which gave rise to an imperfect embryo. Occasionally, fragmentation may be due to poor culture conditions—but only if all the patient's embryos, as well as all other patients' embryos cultured under the same conditions, fragment. If only some embryos fragment, and other patients' embryos appear intact, the problem then lies with the individual embryos themselves.

For diagnostic purposes, it might sometimes be desirable to schedule the transfer in two stages. For example, if 20 eggs were retrieved from a 38-year-old patient with unexplained infertility, and 18 fertilized, the doctor might transfer four on day 3 (at the 6 to 8 cell stage) and then observe the remainder. If the additional observation period showed the couple's embryos to be incapable of surviving past the 12 to 16 cell stage, poor embryo quality could be responsible for the couple's otherwise unexplained infertility. If this were to occur repeatedly, the doctor might advise them to consider using donor eggs. If some of the reserved embryos did go on to become blastocysts, the doctor could either perform a secondary transfer on day 6 or the couple could elect to have the additional embryos cryopreserved at the blastocyst stage for future use. Since the implantation rate markedly decreases as a woman grows older, if the patient is 38 years of age or older, a secondary transfer would probably be the best option.

Some recent data suggest that *all* embryo transfers should be delayed for 5 to 6 days to "weed out" many genetically poor embryos. Transfer of blastocysts only will provide a much higher pregnancy rate per embryo transfer. Yet, the percentage of patients reaching transfer is greatly reduced. Perhaps blastocyst transfer will become the standard practice in the future. Until then, when you compare success rates between IVF clinics, be sure to find out when the majority of embryo transfers take place. Otherwise, you may find yourself comparing "apples and oranges."

The Procedure

Transferring embryos into a woman's uterine cavity is the easiest element of IVF, but it is also the most critical. Abdominal ultrasound may be used to visualize the transfer, since precise placement cannot be assured unless the doctor can see the exact location of the catheter as it is inserted and watch the embryos as they are deposited into the uterus. Otherwise, the embryos could become transferred too low down in the uterus—or they might not make it into the uterine cavity at all.

The patient starts out with a mildly full bladder, which is necessary for a good abdominal ultrasound picture. The doctor inserts a speculum into the woman's vagina and cleans her cervix. A plastic tube is then passed through the woman's cervix into the lower part of the uterine cavity. The embryologist picks up the embryos in the smallest amount of fluid (transfer medium) possible and brings them into the procedure room. The catheter is threaded through the outer plastic tubing the doctor has inserted and is advanced 1/2 to 3/4 inch behind the outer sheath. The embryos are then gently injected into the uterine cavity. Since air bubbles in the transfer medium can be seen via ultrasound, it is actually possible to watch the placement of the embryos on the video monitor.

After placement, the catheter must be removed slowly and gently, since too-rapid removal would create suction that could draw the embryos out of the uterus. Once the catheter has been withdrawn, the embryologist checks it under the microscope to make sure that none of the embryos have stuck to its plastic surface. Should this happen (a rare occurrence) they would be returned to the uterus—but in a lower position so as not to interfere with those embryos that have already been transferred.

After the Transfer

Every couple undergoing IVF needs to understand that it is virtually impossible for the embryos to "fall out" of the uterine cavity due to insufficient rest following the transfer. The implantation process is totally out of the couple's control; if an embryo fails to implant, the cause is almost certainly genetic rather than mechanical. There is nothing either the doctor or the couple can do to make a genetically abnormal embryo "stick."

Although it is generally recommended that patients rest for 1 to 2 hours after the transfer as well as much as possible the next day, and abstain from sexual intercourse for the subsequent two weeks, there is no hard scientific evidence to back up this advice. In fact, a recent German study compared two groups, each consisting of 1,000 IVF patients: the patients in one group rested for two hours post-transfer, while the other resumed normal activities immediately afterward. Pregnancy rates in the two groups turned out to be identical.

Post-Transfer Medications

After the transfer, the woman will usually be advised to take supplemental progesterone to help the embryo implant. Progesterone can be administered via intramuscular injection, vaginal suppository, or tablets which are taken by mouth. Occasionally, the woman will be instructed to take a small dose of HCG every 3 days to help the ovary produce additional progesterone. Supplemental HCG can stimulate ovarian hyperstimulation syndrome and give a false-positive pregnancy test. Since it takes HCG 5 days to be cleared from the body, no pregnancy test should be taken before at least 5 days after the final injection.

THE WAITING PERIOD

We urge patients not to get a pregnancy test until 16 days after the embryo transfer to reduce the probability of false-positives.

Since there is no evidence that bed rest affects the probability of conception, the time will pass much more quickly if the woman remains active and productive during this period. Both partners should do whatever they can to reduce their stress levels and focus on other elements in their lives during this period.

Although every couple needs to decide for themselves whether to tell friends and family about their infertility treatment, many women who have gone through the process report that a significant source of stress during the two-week post-transfer period comes from well-meaning friends and family members who call to ask "how things are going." Even if the couple has been successful in refocusing their own attentions during this period, the well-meaning interest of others may keep bringing them right back to obsessing about whether or not the woman has conceived.

One option for couples who choose to discuss their treatment with others is to do so only in general terms, without divulging the exact dates of procedures. This may save them the stress of having to respond, over and over, to such questions as "Do you feel pregnant?" or "Did you get your period yet?"

IF IVF IS NOT SUCCESSFUL

In deciding what course of action to recommend to couples who have had an unsuccessful IVF cycle, the doctor needs to take into account the woman's age, her response to the medication, the quality and fertilization rate of her eggs, whether any embryos reached the blastocyst stage, and whether the couple has had any embryos frozen for future use. Based on this information, the doctor may suggest either additional IVF cycles or a different course of action. The couple then needs to consider the doctor's recommendation in terms of their own financial and emotional reserves, along with their level of commitment to the goal of creating a biological child.

NEW TECHNOLOGY: IMMATURE OOCYTES IN IVF

There has been a recent flurry of interest in a new IVF technique that calls for the retrieval of immature oocytes from the ovary. The woman takes no fertility drugs; instead, the retrieval is performed right after the woman's menstrual period (day 6 to 9 of her cycle) and the oocytes are incubated in culture media and allowed to mature in the laboratory. Any eggs that reach Metaphase II are injected with sperm via ICSI, and the resulting embryos are transferred in the usual manner. To prepare the lining of her uterus, the woman would take estrogen after the retrieval and then switch to progesterone 2 to 3 days before the transfer.

Since this method eliminates the cost of medication and monitoring, it is very appealing. Unfortunately, since only four babies conceived via this method have been born to date, it may not be a viable option. For one thing, immature follicles (which measure only 4 to 10 mm.) are much more difficult to aspirate from the ovary—except in women with polycystic ovarian syndrome, whose ovaries contain large supplies of follicles in the resting state. Perhaps this technique will prove useful for these women, who typically do not respond well to stimulation, and for women who either cannot or choose not to take fertility drugs. The majority of infertile couples, however, should not pin their hopes on this new methodology.

In Vitro Fertilization: Caroline and Joe

Caroline, a 34-year-old anesthesiologist, had been trying to conceive for 3 years. She has never given birth, but had an early, uncomplicated abortion at age 20. Her diagnostic workup was completely normal but her husband, Joe, 47, was found to have a very low sperm count, with abnormally shaped sperm and poor post-processing velocity. He was never able to father a child, despite having tried for many years during a previous marriage. The working diagnosis for the couple was severe male-factor infertility. Since Joe's sperm was so poor, the doctor advised the couple to skip IUI and IPI and proceed directly to IVF with ICSI. They agreed.

During their first IVF cycle, Caroline responded well to stimulation with Lupron and Fertinex and produced 14, mature-looking eggs. But when the embryologist stripped the eggs to prepare them for ICSI, they were all found to be in Metaphase I and too immature to be fertilized, despite the fact that HCG had been given 44 hours earlier. The eggs were allowed additional time to mature in the lab, but only four went on to reach Metaphase II. The rest never completed maturation. The embryologist performed ICSI on the four mature eggs, but only one embryo developed. This embryo was able to reach only the 6-cell stage before the transfer, and there was also some fragmentation. Sadly, Caroline did not become pregnant.

Although Joe had always believed that he bore the sole responsibility for the couple's failure to conceive, it now appeared that an underlying problem with Caroline's eggs might also be to blame. The doctor advised the couple to repeat IVF in several months with a slightly altered stimulation protocol, to see if the quality of Caroline's eggs could be improved. If the same problem were to occur on the second try, and if the couple remained committed to trying for a pregnancy, he would suggest that they consider IVF with donor eggs.

SUMMARY

IVF is the ultimate diagnostic tool available today. It provides a firsthand look at your eggs and embryos, in order to find any subtle or unanticipated problems on a cellular level. The procedure provides the best opportunity to diagnose what might be otherwise undetectable causes for your infertility. At the same time, IVF is the only diagnostic procedure that gives a couple a chance to conceive at the same time.

With the development of ICSI, the treatment of male infertility has been revolutionized. Even men who produce only the smallest numbers of sperm now have the chance to achieve fatherhood.

Since IVF (with or without ICSI) works best in couples in which the woman is as close to her "biological prime" as possible, don't let anyone try to convince you that you are too young for these techniques. Withholding these most potent and direct cures for infertility in the mistaken belief that a relatively young couple should work toward a "natural" conception is both illogical and counterproductive. IVF is a safe, non-invasive procedure that can help you conceive by bypassing tubal disorders, ovulation problems, and many other sources of unexplained infertility.

CHAPTER 9

STEP 5:

*In Vitro Fertilization (IVF)
With Donor Eggs*

The unfortunate truth is that the age of the potential mother is the single most important factor in predicting the likelihood of success in any infertility treatment. Beyond a certain age, which is different for every woman, the eggs will have genetically deteriorated to such an extent that conception becomes impossible. This point in time usually occurs 5 to 10 years before the onset of menopause, while the woman still gets regular periods and has low FSH levels. When that begins to happen, IVF with donor eggs may offer the only chance for a pregnancy.

The chances for fertilization, implantation, and pregnancy are quite high with donor eggs, because the donors are generally young—between the ages of 18 and 30—and the DNA of eggs produced by such young women is usually intact. In fact, since donor eggs are generally of such high quality, there is a rather low rate of miscarriage among women who use them to conceive.

It may take awhile to get used to the idea of attempting conception with eggs that are genetically unrelated to you. But there are a few important points to consider before you make up your mind. Unlike a woman who adopts, the woman who has conceived via a donor egg actually gives birth to the baby, which makes her the biologic and legal parent. The only record of the egg donation is contained in the files kept by the fertility clinic. Since these files cannot be released without written consent, confidentiality is assured. People who see you pregnant will never think to question the source of the eggs that were responsible for getting you that way. And judging from our experience, once you have held your very own, precious baby in your arms, the source of the eggs won't matter to you, either.

THE DONOR

Donor Recruitment

When a couple elects to use egg donation for an IVF cycle, they may either choose a donor known to them—a friend or relative—or select an anonymous donor.

Women choose to become anonymous egg donors for a variety of reasons. Some have no current interest in becoming pregnant and feel that their eggs are "going to waste." Others donate for truly altruistic purposes, wanting to help couples who are desperate to conceive. Many donors have friends or relatives who are infertile and feel great empathy with the heartache of couples in similar situations. But whatever their motivation, egg donors provide a truly priceless gift to couples who have nowhere else to turn in their quest for a pregnancy. And because there is some inconvenience and potential discomfort associated with taking the required medication, being monitored, and undergoing the retrieval, donors typically receive financial compensation, which is provided by the infertile couple, for their services.

Anonymous egg donors are usually recruited by the doctor's office or infertility clinic via word-of-mouth or through newspaper ads (particularly in college papers). Although the recipient couple gets to learn a great deal about the donor's health, family history, ethnic background, education, and interests, her identity is kept secret. Likewise, the donor never learns the identity of the couples who receive her eggs.

Donor Screening

Before she undergoes medical screening, a potential donor typically goes through an extensive interview process to determine if she is truly motivated to comply with all the requirements that go along with becoming an egg donor. Women who are only interested in the compensation are usually not selected, since experience has shown them to be unreliable.

Donors are also screened for:

- Sexually transmitted diseases
  - Various types of the HIV virus
  - Hepatitis A, B, and C
  - Syphillis
  - Gonorrhea
- Genetically transmitted diseases, where appropriate
  - Sickle cell anemia
  - Tay Sachs disease
- Family history of depression, suicide, or alcohol abuse

As long as these tests are properly performed, IVF with donor eggs poses practically no risk for transmitting infectious diseases to either the mother or newborn.

Even with negative results on all screening tests, some couples may still be concerned about the possibility of contracting AIDS via egg donation. Actually, the process of egg donation is far less apt to transmit disease than is sperm donation. The HIV virus has never been known to affect a developing egg in its follicle. Moreover, donor eggs are obtained by needle puncture and then quickly placed in biologically pure medium—a process that limits potential contact with the donor's blood. Sperm, however, exist in the seminal fluid, which normally contains white blood cells that can harbor the HIV virus. The HIV virus is also known to be able to survive on the surface of the sperm itself, so that washing the sperm does not guarantee immunity from HIV infection.

It is important to know if any of the donor's family members suffer (or have suffered) from such illnesses as depression or alcohol abuse, or if there is a history of suicide, since these personality traits are thought to be inheritable. Family histories of diabetes, heart problems, and cancer are relatively common in our society, and since the role of heredity in their development is uncertain, recipients should probably not reject a potential donor based only on the incidence of one of these diseases in the family tree. In fact, these diseases are so widespread that almost everyone has the potential to develop at least one in their lifetime, regardless of family history—particularly if they don't take care of themselves. Besides, medical science has developed excellent screening and treatment techniques for many of these illnesses, so even if the baby does go on to develop one of them in middle age, he or she can still go on to live a long, active life.

Selecting A Donor

Traditionally, sperm banks have never provided recipients with photographs of potential donors. This leaves a lot to the imagination.

We feel strongly that recipients will feel more comfortable with the entire process if photographs of potential donors are available for them to view when they make their selection. Patients in our clinic look through binders containing anonymous photos of potential donors, along with information on the donor's age, ethnic background, religion, physical attributes (height, weight, complexion, eye and hair color, hair texture), education, occupation, and special interests. In our experience, the closer the egg donor's resemblance to the mother in terms of physical appearance and genetic background, the better the experience will be. Therefore, couples are encouraged to select a donor whose face bears some resemblance to the mother. This also helps to minimize concern by the potential parents that outsiders will guess that the baby is not the mother's genetic offspring.

"Should We Tell?"

One of the most common questions by potential recipient couples is whether they should tell friends, family, and ultimately, the child, that the conception was achieved via donor eggs.

Ultimately, each couple must decide for themselves whether or not to share the details of their child's conception. However, we advise couples who are leaning toward disclosure to at least wait until after the baby is born to share the information with others. Once a woman has carried a baby for nine months and then gone through childbirth, the origin of the egg usually becomes truly irrelevant.

If a couple does decide to tell, they should follow an "all-or-nothing" rule. If even one other person knows about the egg donation, there will always be the possibility that their confidentiality will be violated. Regardless of their ultimate decision, the couple's obstetrician should be told about the donation, since the fact that the egg comes from a younger woman is relevant to the decision as to whether or not amniocentesis should be performed. Couples can request that this information not be placed in the woman's medical record.

Donor Sharing

In almost all donor egg programs, the donor's oocytes are shared between two recipient couples, the identities of whom are kept secret from each other. There are many benefits to this practice. Many times a donor produces too many embryos for one couple to use. If the recipient couple conceives on the first try, the additional embryos, which have been frozen for future attempts, tend to go unused. This is truly wasteful of one of the most precious of human resources. On a more practical note, sharing donor oocytes reduces the recipient couple's waiting time—which may be several months or more at some clinics—and expense. Each recipient couple must now only pay for half of the donor's medication costs and fee, which can result in a saving of some $3000.

Even with sharing, each couple usually receives three-to-six embryos, some of which can be frozen for later use if the initial attempt should fail.

THE PROCEDURE

The Recipient

The first step in the egg donation process is to synchronize the menstrual cycles of donor and recipient. This is most easily accomplished when the recipient is either post-menopausal or does not get her periods for some other reason. These patients are typically placed on estrogen until the endometrium develops to 9 to 12 mm—a level which can be detected on a sonogram. The endometrium can be kept in that state for 6 to 8 weeks while the donor is prepared for stimulation.

Since pregnancy rates with donor eggs seem to be higher for women who do not menstruate, potential recipients who do still get their periods can be given a "pseudo-menopause" through the use of Depot (long-acting) Lupron. The recipient will receive an injection of 3.75 mg of Depot Lupron on day 1 to 5 of her period, and this will be repeated every 30 days. Usually, she needs only 2 to 3 shots before her period disappears. She will then be given estrogen to produce a thick, lush endometrium for her potential embryos. Estrogen can be administered via pill (4 to 6 mg Estrace per day), patch (4 to 6 patches changed every other day) or injection (4 to 6 mg every 3 to 4 days). The recipient is kept in endometrial readiness while the donor is stimulated.

The Donor

The protocol for the donor is similar to the recipient in terms of suppression of her natural cycle. She receives an injection of Depot Lupron between days 1 and 5 of her menstrual cycle; the shot is repeated thirty days thereafter. After the second Lupron injection the donor can be stimulated with gonadotropins for a period of up to 3 to 4 weeks. The donor is monitored during her stimulation and the recipient is kept informed of her progress.

Pre- and Post-Transfer

When the donor is ready to receive her HCG and the egg retrieval is 36 to 38 hours away, the recipient and her husband are notified. The male partner is told when to come to the office on the day of the retrieval to produce a sperm specimen, while the recipient needs to receive an intramuscular injection of 100 mg of progesterone to help prepare her endometrium. The progesterone injection is repeated for 2 or more days, and the transfer is performed on the third or fourth day thereafter. Usually, only 3 to 4 embryos are transferred, and the remainder (if any) are frozen for either a subsequent cycle or, if the first transfer is successful, a second child. The transfer procedure itself is the same as for a standard IVF cycle.

After the transfer, the recipient takes a progesterone supplement for the next 16 days. The progesterone can be administered either via intramuscular injection, vaginal suppositories, or tablets. The recipient's blood progesterone levels are monitored on an occasional basis so that the dosage can be adjusted as necessary. Ideally, the recipient's blood level of progesterone should be more than15 nanograms/ml on the third day post-transfer.

In many instances, the progesterone supplementation associated with donor oocytes delays the recipient's period. Since we don't want patients to feel falsely encouraged—only to get their hopes dashed if a 14-day pregnancy test proves negative—we urge recipients to wait 16 days after the transfer before getting a pregnancy test.

IF A DONOR CYCLE IS SUCCESSFUL

A woman who conceives via donor eggs should be monitored via blood hormone level testing and ultrasound 2 weeks after a positive pregnancy test. At that time, it should be possible to determine the number of viable fetuses.

Normally, once a woman has conceived via donor eggs she is no more at risk for complications than any other pregnant woman. Routine amniocentesis is not called for, since the age of the donor (usually under 30), rather than the age of the recipient, is the relevant factor in assessing the chances for genetic abnormality of the fetus. We advise blood testing at 15 weeks as a non-invasive means of screening for Down's Syndrome and neural defects such as spina bifida. If the results of these tests are normal, the mother does not need to undergo amniocentesis, as the risk of a resulting miscarriage would be greater than the risk of the child bearing a chromosomal abnormality.

The only other increased risks for a woman pregnant via donor eggs are related to age. An older woman going through pregnancy might have a higher-than-normal chance of developing such age-related complications as high blood pressure (pre-eclampsia) or gestational diabetes; however, all women are routinely screened for these conditions during pregnancy. It is not usually necessary to select an obstetrician who specializes in high-risk pregnancies unless a preexisting medical condition exists or if a complication develops during the pregnancy.

IF A DONOR CYCLE IS NOT SUCCESSFUL

Just as with one's own eggs, achieving a pregnancy with donor eggs is usually a matter of persistence. However, if a particular donor's eggs don't produce a pregnancy after two or three attempts (despite good stimulation and the production of a large number of eggs), the couple should switch to a different donor. The clinic should probably terminate this donor's participation in the program, since the genetic quality of her eggs may have already started to deteriorate. For their second donor, the couple might be well-advised to select a woman whose eggs have created a recent pregnancy.

IVF With Donor Eggs: Caroline and Joe

Caroline and Joe, the couple who had unsuccessfully attempted IVF in Chapter 8, remained unable to conceive despite two additional IVF cycles. The doctor urged them to consider donor eggs. Joe was extremely eager to become a father, so he readily agreed. Caroline was a little more reluctant about the fact that she would be carrying a child with whom she would have no genetic tie. She admitted to being afraid that she would feel as though she were "carrying someone else's baby." But she was desperate to experience pregnancy, and she knew how much Joe wanted a child, so she finally acquiesced.

The first donor that Caroline and Joe selected looked very much like Caroline, with a similar ethnic background. Unfortunately, the donor produced only two eggs, neither of which fertilized. The couple decided to try once more, but this time with a different donor. For this cycle, they selected a woman who looked less like Caroline but whose eggs had been successfully used in a previous cycle with a different patient. Although this donor did not resemble Caroline, she and Joe liked the doctor's description of the donor's personality.

"She has a wonderful smile, and she lights up whatever room she's in," he told the couple.

This donor produced nine mature oocytes, five of which were allocated to Caroline. Thanks to ICSI, Joe's sperm fertilized four of the eggs, all of which were successfully transferred to Caroline's uterus. After three weeks, Caroline learned she was pregnant.

When their son, Matthew, was born 9 months later, Caroline and Joe were overjoyed. Caroline admitted that once she had experienced morning sickness, felt the baby kick, seen his image in her sonograms, and grown to love the feel of him inside her womb, the lack of a genetic tie with her son had become completely irrelevant. The couple never told anyone about having used an egg donor, and to the best of their knowledge, no one in the family suspected that Matthew was anyone other than Caroline's own son, in every way possible.

DONOR CYTOPLASM AUGMENTATION: A GLIMMER OF HOPE ON THE FAR HORIZON

Some doctors have theorized that the deterioration of the cytoplasm, which is the complex gel that surrounds the DNA-containing nucleus of the egg, may be responsible for the increased conception failures and higher rates of miscarriage experienced by older women. Since the spindle mechanism—the body on which the chromosomes of the egg and sperm are arranged for distribution during the course of fertilization—is contained in the cytoplasm, it appears logical that deterioration of certain components of the cytoplasm may be a serious impediment to conception.

Very recently, the first successful attempt to correct a potential cytoplasmic problem was announced in the media. News reports touted the birth of a baby whose conception was attributed to doctors having supplemented the cytoplasm in the mother's own egg with a small amount of cytoplasm from a donor egg. Thus, although a donor egg was involved in the conception, the actual genetic material came from the mother rather than the donor. And since the couple's three previous IVF attempts had failed, the conception was credited to the addition of donor cytoplasm during ICSI.

Although these reports may provide new hope to infertile couples who reject the idea of conception via donor eggs, a degree of caution would be wise. First, the news item came about as a result of a letter-to-the-editor of a well-known medical journal, rather than from a scientific research paper. Although everyone is understandably excited, a scientific or medical technique cannot be judged effective on the basis of one single anecdotal case report. Just by mere chance, this particular patient could have conceived because a genetically perfect egg had been united with a perfect sperm (she had responded well to the fertility drugs and had produced many eggs during this cycle). In addition, no one knows for sure whether the tiny bit of cytoplasm transferred to her egg contained some essential component which contributed to the conception.

Hopefully, donor cytoplamic augmentation will provide a solution to some patients' problems. But before we can make an informed decision about the utility of this potentially exciting technique, it needs to be scientifically proven via the appropriate research methodology. Several hundred patients matched by age and clinical history should be evaluated, with half of the group receiving cytoplasmic augmentation and the other half having normal IVF with ICSI. Only if the study produces positive results that are statistically significant will we be able to endorse the procedure with complete confidence.

SUMMARY

If deteriorating eggs or a diminished egg supply are keeping you from becoming pregnant, donor eggs may offer you a realistic hope. Pregnancy rates with donor eggs are high, and when properly coordinated, the procedure is relatively easy. You will still have the opportunity to experience pregnancy, and should you decide not to tell anyone about the circumstances of your baby's conception, no one need ever know.

Donor eggs can make pregnancy a reality for couples whose only other choice may be adoption.

C H A P T E R   1 0

WHAT ABOUT THE UTERUS?

The question of whether to follow the success- or diagnosis-oriented approach is by no means the only controversy associated with infertility treatment. Another subject widely open to debate is whether certain conditions in the uterus can cause infertility by preventing new embryos from implanting. The question is relevant both to embryos created naturally and to those created via IVF and donor eggs.

The three factors most commonly blamed for rendering a uterus "unreceptive" are:

1. Inadequate progesterone levels

2. Abnormal physical structure of the woman's endometrium (uterine lining)

3. Inappropriate responses to the developing embryo by the mother's immune system

PROGESTERONE LEVELS

After ovulation, the progesterone produced by the ovary prepares the endometrium for an embryo to implant on the 6 to 7th day following the release of the egg. It is well known from the early days of IVF, though, that embryos can implant as early as two days after ovulation, since all transfers used to be performed at that time. We also know from our own experience that the endometrium actually requires only minimal exposure to progesterone in order for pregnancy to occur.

Inadequate Progesterone: Maria

Maria, a hispanic patient with only a limited understanding of English, was scheduled for IVF with donor eggs. In preparation for the embryo transfer, she had received an intramuscular injection of 100 mg of progesterone on the day of the donor's retrieval. The doctor gave her two 100 mg oral progesterone tablets and told her to take one (by mouth!) each day prior to the transfer. But unbeknownst to the doctor or office staff, Maria did not understand the instructions. Instead of swallowing the tablets, she inserted them into her vagina. Since oral tablets are not meant to be inserted intravaginally, little of the progesterone was absorbed into Maria's system. The mistake was discovered at the time of the transfer, when the doctor noticed residue from the tablets on the walls of her vagina.

Since this happened before the technology for cryopreserving (preserving via freezing) had been perfected, the doctor had no choice but to transfer the embryos anyway, despite the fact that her progesterone level was only 5.0 ng/ml, rather than the desired 15-or-more ng/ml. Amazingly, three out of the five embryos implanted, and Maria became pregnant with triplets!

Since IVF pregnancy rates have been shown to be highest when the embryo transfer takes place 3 to 6 days after the egg retrieval, we hold off on the transfer until that time. We don't know, however, if these success rates are due to the increased maturity of the uterine lining or to the advanced development of the embryo itself.

In IVF, when a woman's progesterone levels rise prematurely (before her eggs are ready to be retrieved), it is of greater concern than potentially inadequate progesterone. If the rise in progesterone begins too early, it means that the woman's period may also start too early. If we were to transfer any embryos during that cycle, the premature menstrual flow would be certain to wash tham away. Our only option would be to cryopreserve (freeze) the embryos for transfer during a subsequent cycle.

STRUCTURAL ABNORMALITIES

The role of the uterine lining in implantation failure is uncertain. Since embryos have been known to implant where no endometrial tissue exists at all, i.e., in the Fallopian tubes (in ectopic pregnancies), on the surface of the ovaries, and even in the abdominal cavity, we believe the "receptivity" of the uterus is relatively unimportant. However, the chances for pregnancy will probably be best when the recipient has a structurally sound, well-developed endometrium (10 to 12 mm). Structure appears to be more important than thickness. In fact, we have seen pregnancies in women with uterine linings that were only 6 mm in thickness, but were well formed into its three layers.

Before the embryo transfer, if the patient is found to have a very thin, dense endometrium, one that is thick (>15 mm) and "spongy," or a lining that does not consist of the three well-developed layers, we would probably advise freezing the embryos for a future cycle in which the endometrium had a more normal appearance. For subsequent cycles, we would help the patient develop a cleaner uterine lining by changing the type of estrogen we prescribed.

On the rare occasion that a woman's endometrium does not respond whatsoever to estrogen stimulation, it might mean that there is scar tissue inside the uterus. In those cases—or if the doctor feels it would be helpful to "freshen" a thick, spongy endometrium—a D&C (a minor surgical procedure in which the uterine lining can be scraped clean) might be helpful in stimulating the growth of a better endometrium.

Two other uterine conditions that could make a woman a poor candidate for embryo transfer are multiple fibroids in the cavity of the uterus, and a condition known as adenomyosis, in which endometriosis-like tissue is present in the muscular layer of the uterus. If a woman with either of these conditions has had multiple failures of donor embryo transfers, she should probably abandon further attempts to conceive. And since fibroids >10 mm located inside the uterine cavity can be associated with late first trimester miscarriage, such fibroids should probably be surgically removed before the embryo transfer is attempted.

HYDROSALPINX: ITS POTENTIAL FOR ADVERSE EFFECTS ON THE UTERUS

When a woman is found to have fluid in her Fallopian tubes, the condition is called hydrosalpinx. At present, there is substantial evidence that the tubal fluid in women with hydrosalpinx leaks back into the uterus. This brings substances to the endometrium that are toxic to the embryo, preventing implantation. In this way, hydrosalpinx may adversely affect the outcome of IVF.

There are two ways to prevent hydrosalpinx from interfering with the IVF process: either the tube(s) can be surgically removed, or the fluid can be drained from the tube prior to the embryo transfer. Although surgical removal of the tube can usually be accomplished via minimally invasive laparoscopic surgery (occasionally an abdominal incision becomes necessary), the procedure still requires general anesthesia, carries the associated risks, and requires a certain recovery period. Our personal preference is the less invasive method, which is to drain the tubes at the time of the egg retrieval. After the eggs are removed from the ovary, the same needle is passed into the dilated Fallopian tube and the fluid contained inside is aspirated. In our experience, after the tube has been drained the fluid does not reaccumulate for several weeks, at which time it should not adversely affect a successful pregnancy. However, if a sonogram proved it necessary, we would drain the tube a second time prior to the embryo transfer.

If a hydrosalpinx contained only a minimal amount of fluid, we would probably not take surgical action unless the couple had 2 to 3 unsuccessful IVF cycles in which excellent quality embryos were transferred and age was not a factor. In these cases, we would recommend laparoscopic removal of the tubes.

IMMUNOLOGY AND INFERTILITY

The job of the human immune system is to recognize and destroy foreign ("nonself") organisms that invade the body (bacteria, viruses, etc.). While it is meant to protect us from disease, this important defense system may also cause harm—for example, when it causes the body to reject a transplanted organ or attacks it s own tissue, as in autoimmune diseases.

The role of the immune system in infertility is difficult to evaluate and subject to much debate. Some physicians speculate that, in certain women, the immune system perceives a developing embryo or fetus as foreign tissue and rejects it just as it would a transplanted liver or heart. These physicians blame immunologic mechanisms for the high numbers of early miscarriages and IVF implantation failures. They say that the placenta usually constructs an immunologic barrier which protects the fetus from the body's defense system, and that a breakdown in the barrier can cause pregnancy losses at all stages.

Infertility specialists who believe the immune system has a role in causing pregnancy loss treat IVF implantation failures as "early," recurrent miscarriages. Such doctors typically perform an extensive battery of tests on their patients for immunologic substances such as: embryotoxic factors; antithyroid antibodies; antiphospholipids and anticardiolipin antibodies; "natural killer lymphocytes"; anti DNA antibodies; and HLA (human leukocyte antigens—the transplantation antigens). Based on the results of these tests, the doctor might offer therapies ranging from the relatively benign—such as treatment with low-dose aspirin or heparin (a blood thinner)—to the more complex—e.g., the transfer of paternal white blood cells to the woman, treatment with high-dose corticosteroids, or IVIG, which is intravenous therapy with gamma globulin (mixed blood products).

There is no hard scientific evidence to prove the efficacy of treatments for these supposed immune system disorders. In one such treatment—the transfer of paternal leukocytes—four out of five randomized studies showed that the treatment had no beneficial effect over performing no treatment at all. Another study of 800 patients showed that elevated antiphospholipid antibody levels were not associated with any change in pregnancy rates or pregnancy loss rates in patients attempting to conceive via IVF. Yet, physicians offer these treatments without explaining that they are considered experimental.

Doctors who disagree with the immunologic theory blame the relatively high rate of early miscarriage and IVF failures on genetic abnormalities, which they believe to be nature's way of protecting the species. They believe that any pregnancy loss in which there has been no fetal development is actually a *genetic* loss due to a poor quality egg (known as a blighted ovum). Only a pregnancy loss in which the fetus has attained a heartbeat and experienced normal development of the other organ systems (this usually occurs by the tenth week) can be considered anything but a genetic loss. If a healthy pregnancy grows and develops past the twelfth week, but then either dies or starts to lose growth, only then should an immunological cause be considered. However, a pregnancy loss at this stage could also be due to a twisted umbilical cord or an intrauterine infection.

Immunologic Problems?: Norma and Bob

Norma was 33-years-old and had never been pregnant, despite the fact that she and her husband, Bob, had used no birth control for the entire twelve years they had been together.

A little more than one year ago, the couple consulted an immunologist. Norma was diagnosed as having an immunologic problem which required that she be immunized (injected) with her husband's white blood cells. This treatment continued for 1 year, but the couple did not conceive.

Norma and Bob then requested an IVF cycle. The immunologist prescribed Heparin (a blood thinner) therapy as an adjunct to the IVF treatment. Norma had very good stimulation and produced twelve follicles with high estradiol levels. However during the retrieval, the doctor was surprised to learn that Norma had really produced only five eggs; the rest of the follicles were empty. Of the five eggs, only two were normal. They went on to fertilize, and the two embryos were transferred. Unfortunately, Norma did not become pregnant.

The results of her IVF cycle proved that instead of suffering from an exotic and rare immunologic problem, Norma had a simple and straightforward egg problem. This supports our opinion that getting pregnant is easy with good eggs. If a woman is not getting pregnant—although everything appears "normal"—she should assume that her eggs are to blame, and she should think twice before resorting to expensive immunologic testing and risky immunologic therapy.

Although some physicians do report good results from immunologic treatments, the question always remains whether the treatment was responsible for a pregnancy or whether that particular embryo just happened to be genetically sound and in the appropriate position for survival. Moreover, there are countless documented cases of women with numerous miscarriages who go on to achieve normal pregnancies without any intervention (immunologic or otherwise) whatsoever. Even women with high levels of antithyroid antibodies (which have been shown to double a woman's risk of miscarriage) have gone on to have successful pregnancies without treatment.

Immunologic testing and treatment add significant expense to a couple's infertility treatment. A course of therapy with IV gammaglobulin may cost as much as $12,000. Some treatments may also carry a significant degree of risk—particularly during the transfer of blood products, which can potentially transfer certain viruses to the woman, and during treatment with high doses of corticosteroids, which can cause significant mental and physical side effects.

When a Patient Gets Too Much Advice: Lisa

Lisa was a 41-year-old woman who had been trying to become pregnant for 2 years. During her first IVF attempt, seven eggs were retrieved. Although three went on to become fertilized, she did not conceive. On her second IVF attempt, Lisa produced ten eggs—six of which fertilized. One of those embryos successfully implanted, and Lisa was ecstatic about her pregnancy. She told everyone she knew, and friends and family were delighted. Unfortunately, ultrasound monitoring showed abnormal development of the fetal sac, which meant that the pregnancy had been created from an abnormal egg. Within 3 weeks, Lisa had miscarried.

Understandably shattered, Lisa turned to those closest to her for advice. On the recommendation of her younger sister, Lisa logged onto the Internet to see what she could learn about infertility and pregnancy loss. She happened upon the home page of an infertility expert who strongly believed immune system disorders to be the cause of most early miscarriages. Since the doctor's practice was nearby, she made an appointment for a consultation. On the basis of that discussion, Lisa and her husband decided to suspend their infertility treatment for 6 months to undergo the extensive immunologic testing and treatment that the doctor was recommending.

Whether or not Lisa will conceive remains to be seen. But even if she does succeed after her intensive immunologic workup, the cause of her infertility will remain far from certain. During the first trimester, women over the age of 40 have a 50 to 70 percent chance of miscarriage due to early genetic abnormalities of fetal development. This is completely apart from any potential immunologic effect. If Lisa conceives after her immunologic treatment, we will never know if that was responsible, or if she finally just "got a good egg."

SUMMARY

At Advanced Fertility Services, we believe that the rejection of "early embryos" is entirely genetic. We hesitate to recommend diagnostic tests and treatments that serve to increase the expense and risk associated with infertility treatment without providing proven results.

Infertility patients are desperate to "do something" to alter their condition, but sometimes it is necessary to just wait the problem out, instead of spending significant amounts of time and money on questionable testing and treatment. Although the heartbreak of miscarriage causes severe emotional pain—particularly if pregnancy has been difficult to achieve—we try to help couples understand that it is not always possible to find an answer as to why things happen. We urge them to trust in nature and believe that whatever happens, happens for a reason—even if we can't always see it at the time.

CHAPTER 11

HOW MUCH IS ALL THIS GOING TO COST?

There's no way around it—infertility treatment is not cheap. The costs of the procedures and medications can seem daunting—especially when you're just starting out. But before you panic, don't forget that you need to balance the costs associated with whatever treatment you select against the likelihood that it will result in a pregnancy. Don't be scared off by procedures like IVF that seem to be expensive at first, since in the long run, they may provide both important diagnostic information and quicker, more reliable results, making them more cost-effective on an overall basis.

Here are some average costs for the individual procedures and treatments we've described. These are based on the fee schedule currently in place at Advanced Fertility Services in New York City (obviously, costs will vary by by center and by geographic location). Later on in the chapter, we'll compare the costs of complete courses of success-oriented treatment versus. diagnosis-oriented treatment in some couples, and discuss insurance coverage.

COSTS

Traditional Diagnostic Workup

FOR HER:

Initial consultation	$	250.
Physical exam	$	100.
Cervical cultures	$	120.
Anti-chlamydia antibody test	$	60.
Blood hormone level tests		
FSH	$	80.
LH	$	80.
Estradiol	$	80.
TSH	$	80.
T_3	$	80.
T_4	$	80.
Prolactin	$	80.
DEAS	$	80.
Progesterone	$	80.
Total	**$**	**720.**
At-home urine ovulation test	$	40. each
Pelvic sonogram	$	150.
Hysterosalpingogram (HSG)	$	450.
Post-coital test (PCT)	$	100.
Endometrial biopsy	$	400.
Laparoscopy		
Procedure	$	2,000.
Anesthesia	$	1,500.
Hospital	$	2,500.
Total	**$**	**6,000.**

TOTAL COST OF WORKUP FOR HER: **$ 8,390.**

FOR HIM:

Initial consultation	$	*250.*
Physical exam	$	*100.*
Semen analysis	$	*150.*
Hamster test	$	*350.*

TOTAL COST OF WORKUP FOR HIM	$	**850.**

FOR THE COUPLE:

Anti-sperm antibody test	$	*600.*

TOTAL COST OF WORKUP FOR THE COUPLE:	$	**600.**

POTENTIAL TOTAL COST OF A TRADITIONAL WORKUP $ 9,840.

TREATMENT OPTIONS:
Clomiphene citrate + IUI Cycle

Clomiphene citrate:		
$6.00 /tablet X 10 tablets	$	*60.*
Urine ovulation predictor kit	$	*40.*
Sonogram	$	*150.*
Sperm Processing	$	*150.*
IUI	$	*150.*

TOTAL COST PER CYCLE	$	**550.**

Gonadotropin + IPI Cycle

Gonadotropin

  4 amps/day for 9 days

  (Cost/amp: $50.) $ 1,800.

HCG $ 30.

Monitoring

  3 sonograms: $ 450.

  3 blood tests: $ 240.

    Total monitoring: $ 690.

Sperm processing: $ 150.

Follicle Puncture and Insemination: $ 600.

TOTAL COST PER CYCLE: **$ 3,270.**

In Vitro Fertilization Cycle
Cost of a Basic IVF Cycle at AFS Includes:

  Monitoring

  Egg Retrieval

  Culture

  Sperm Preparation

  Embryo Transfer

  Total IVF $ 5,500.

Medication $ 1,500 - 2,500.

ICSI $ 1,000.

Assisted Hatching $ 800.

TOTAL COST PER CYCLE $ **7,000-$9,800.**

The cost of a basic IVF cycle at centers across the country ranges between $4,000 and $12,000. This usually includes monitoring (blood tests and sonograms), egg retrieval, sperm preparation, and the embryo transfer. The necessary medications can add some $1,500 to $2,500 to each cycle. If a couple requires ICSI, the cost per cycle can increase by $1,000, and in some clinics, co-culture can add as much as another $2,000 to the bill. In all, a couple could end up spending more than $15,000 for a single IVF treatment cycle.

The high costs associated with IVF are due to the fact that it is a highly labor-intensive endeavor requiring an extremely high level of quality control. Clinics must be open seven-days-per week, and sophisticated (and expensive) equipment, supplies, and laboratory materials are required. In addition, there are significant administrative costs associated with the data collection that is required by the Society for Advanced Reproductive Techniques, which is the industry's professional organization. Moreover, the fertility medications used in IVF are quite costly, with costs in this country that are more than twice as high as in Europe and South America.

That said, there are certain mitigating factors with regard to the apparently high costs of IVF.

First, IVF centers charge varying fees for their services. A clinic's fee structure will depend upon its location, size, whether the clinic is free-standing or hospital affiliated, and on the number of procedures performed. In general, the more cases per clinic, the lower the cost of an individual cycle will be, since the fixed costs (e.g., equipment, personnel) will be shared among a greater number of patients. In fact, there may be an inverse relationship between cost and quality of care —that is, the clinic that charges the most may actually perform the fewest IVF procedures, giving them the least practical experience. So just as a couple considering IVF should compare the success rates of the various treatment centers they are considering, so should they compare the costs quoted by the facilities.

Also, it may be possible to reduce the costs associated with certain procedures, e.g., sharing a donor egg cycle between two recipients or harvesting sperm for an IVF/ICSI cycle at the same time a testicular biopsy is performed.

And finally, you should be sure to consider *the total cost of your expected treatment* rather than comparing individual charges on a procedure-by-procedure basis. Procedures that initially appear to be expensive, like IVF, may provide quicker, more reliable results than other approaches. In addition, using IVF may allow you to eliminate other expensive but less useful tests and procedures, like diagnostic laparoscopy.

COST COMPARISON: TRADITIONAL VERSUS SUCCESS-ORIENTED TREATMENT

To illustrate the potential differences between traditional and success-oriented treatment, let's compare the total costs of therapy for the couples described in Chapter 2:

Susan and Mark, Diagnosis-oriented method:

Case history/initial evaluation		$ 250.
Cervical cultures		$ 120.
Semen analysis		$ 150.
HSG		$ 450.
Laparoscopy		$ 6,000.
Gonadotropin/IUI (3 cycles)		
IUI;	$ 450.	
Gonadotropins:	$ 5,400.	
Total:		$ 5,850.
Second HSG:		$ 450.
Endometrial biopsy		$ 400.
Two IVF cycles (including medication)		$ 14,000.

TOTAL COST OF CONCEPTION: **$27,670.**

Susan and Mark, Success-oriented method:

Case history/initial evaluation	$ 250.
Anti-chlamydial antibody blood test	$ 60.
Blood Tests (FSH/LH/Estrodiol)	$ 240.
Semen analysis	$ 150.
Sonogram	$ 150.
HSG	$ 450.
Two IVF cycles: (including medication)	$ 14,000.

TOTAL COST OF CONCEPTION: **$15,300.**

**POTENTIAL SAVINGS WITH
SUCCESS-ORIENTED APPROACH:**   **$12,370.**

Kate and Steven, Diagnosis-oriented method:

Case history/initial evaluation		$	250.
Semen analysis		$	150.
HSG		$	450.
Varicocele surgery		$	3,500.
Second semen analysis		$	150.
Gonadotropin/IUI (3 cycles)			
IUI	$ 450.		
Gonadotropins	$ 5,400.		
Total		$	5,850.
Two IVF cycles with ICSI		$	17,000

TOTAL COST OF CONCEPTION: **$27,350.**

Kate and Steven, Success-oriented method:

Case history/initial evaluation	$	250.
Antichlamydial antibody blood test	$	60.
HSG	$	450.
Semen analysis	$	150.
Two IVF cycles with ICSI	$	17,000.

TOTAL COST OF CONCEPTION: **$17,910.**

**POTENTIAL SAVINGS WITH
SUCCESS-ORIENTED APPROACH:**   **$ 9,440.**

The success-oriented approach saved both couples significant amounts of money and time, and made many of the painful and invasive procedures associated with traditional infertility treatment unnecessary. The success-oriented strategy also made evident valuable information about the couples' fertility status early on in the treatment process.

INSURANCE COVERAGE

Some medical insurance policies cover at least some portion of infertility treatment, and some states mandate coverage (only eight states cover IVF). As of 1997, some infertility coverage is mandated in the following states:

Maryland   *Rhode Island*

Ohio   *New York (does not mandate IVF coverage)*

Arkansas

Hawaii   *Illinois*

Massachusetts   *Montana*

West Virginia

In addition, Texas, Connecticut, and California are required to offer infertility insurance.

In other cases, medical insurance will cover some of the costs associated with blood tests, sonograms, and medications. However, most insurance companies have avoided paying for IVF because they feel this will lead to a "bottomless pit" of expenses, and that couples would attempt unreasonable numbers of IVF cycles even after the point that success could be reasonably expected. Recent studies have shown, however, that when

IVF is covered, the cost of an individual insurance policy is increased by less than $2.50 per member, per month.

Many IVF centers have insurance coordinators to help patients determine their potential benefits, and some clinics accept assignment with proper documentation. Such clinics do a great service to patients, since the couple's out-of-pocket expenses will be only a relatively small proportion of the total cost. In any case, couples should try to get a predetermination of benefits from their insurance company in writing before starting treatment with IVF. If your policy does not provide coverage for IVF, it may be possible to purchase an infertility/IVF rider. Finally, bear in mind that insurance policies invariably cover more costs associated with diagnostic tests than for therapeutic procedures.

RESOLVE, the national infertility patient advocacy group, has mounted a strong lobby for a national mandate requiring coverage of infertility treatments. Hopefully, there will soon be additional financial relief for couples undergoing fertility treatment.

SUMMARY

Before you start on any infertility treatment, there are a few questions you need to ask yourself. First of all, do you want to spend the next 1 to 2 years and some $15,000 to $20,000 trying to diagnose and fix whatever is preventing you from having a baby, and then wait to see if the diagnosis was correct enough to allow you to become pregnant? Or would you rather spend less than $2,000 on a limited diagnostic workup and then quickly proceed to the step that is most likely to be successful in your particular situation?

Whichever you decide, it is important to know exactly which portion of your expenses will be covered by your medical insurance policy, and to get a predetermination of benefits in writing. And finally, don't be afraid to "shop around" and compare the prices associated with various approaches and between clinics. As a healthcare consumer, it is your right to do so

CHAPTER TWELVE

WHICH PATH IS RIGHT FOR YOU?

A SUCCESS STORY

O n our third wedding anniversary, my husband and I decided that we were ready, both financially and emotionally, to have a child. We spent almost a year trying to conceive—our lives totally focused on those few days each month when we could plant the seeds for a new life. But they never "took."

Eventually we accepted the fact that if we wanted to have a baby, we would need some help. Since I was already forty-one-years-old, my gynecologist was not encouraging.

"Your eggs are probably no good anymore," he said. "There's not much I can do." Finally, the fertility program in a nearby hospital agreed to take us on. "You'll have to go through our entire treatment protocol," they said. "First we'll see if you're ovulating, and then we'll make sure your tubes are open. It would probably be helpful to take a look inside your belly and see if you have any endometriosis. We'll do some tests to see how well your husband's sperm looks, and we'll make sure you don't have an immune problem. Then if it looks like you will need IVF, you'll have to meet with our psychiatrist and social worker to make sure you and your husband are good candidates for the procedure." The idea of spending all that time on testing made me nervous. The thought of having an operation scared me to death. And when we figured out what the whole process would cost, we both started having second thoughts. "Why don't you just forget trying, and be grateful for what you have," my friends said, when I asked their advice.

Of course I was grateful for the wonderful life I led. But I had so much love to give, and I ached for a baby to share it with.

We finally made our decision. We weren't ready to stop trying for a pregnancy…but I wasn't ready to become a hospital patient, and neither of us was prepared to wade through the mass of tests that had been prescribed. So we found a doctor with another approach—a success-oriented approach. I was lucky enough to develop six eggs on my first IVF cycle. Four of them fertilized, and unbelievably, one of those tiny embryos took hold and survived.

Now, at ten weeks, it still seems like a dream…until we go for our biweekly sonogram. It's only when we see the image of a baby deep inside of me—where before there was only an empty space— that the reality hits. I know that we are truly lucky, but I also know that it was more than just luck that got me pregnant. It was learning which kind of infertility treatment would be right for us and holding out till we found it.

Each time we leave the doctor's office, the sun always seems a little brighter, the day—a little nicer, my life—a little more full.

Our goal for *The Pregnancy Prescription* has been to make you aware of what we believe to be the most *direct, cost-efficient, and time-effective* route to resolving infertility: the success-oriented approach. We've provided step-by-step instructions for following this state-of-the-art plan. But just as there are no guarantees in life, there are also no guarantees in fertility treatment. Should conception prove impossible for you and your partner, please believe that you still have choices. Adoption might provide the answer to your prayers. Or you may honestly come to decide that child-free living is the best choice for you right now.

No one can tell you how your quest for a child will end. We've provided the road map; it's up to you to chart your own journey and to trust in the combination of nature and technology.

We wish you a "success-oriented" journey.

GLOSSARY

acrosome: the package of enzymes at the tip of the sperm that help it penetrate the egg

adenomyosis: the condition in which endometriosis exists in the muscular layer of the uterus

adhesions: two separate surfaces, stuck to each other

aneuploidy: a condition in which an embryo has too much or too little genetic material

antibody: a substance created by one's own immune system to fight off a "foreign" invader, like a bacteria or a virus

antichlamydial antibodies: a substance created by the body to fight infection by the organism, chlamydia, which remains in the body and provides indication of a prior infection

aspirate: the use of suction to remove fluid from a container or from somewhere in the body

assisted hatching: a micromanipulation procedure in which the embryologist thins the zona pellucida of the embryo before it is transferred

autoimmune disease: an illness caused by the body attacking its own tissues

azoospermia: the condition in which a male's semen contains no sperm

basal body temperature (BBT): body temperature at rest, immediately upon awakening. Charting a woman's daily BBT was a common method of determining if ovulation had occurred.

blastocyst: an advanced embryo

blastomere: one of the individual cells that make up an embryo.

chlamydia: an infectious organism which may cause irreparable damage to the Fallopian tubes

cilia: the hairs that line the inner Fallopian tubes

clomiphene citrate: an oral fertility medication (brand names: Clomid, Serophone)

co-culture: living cells that are added to the commercially-produced culture media used in IVF

controlled ovarian hyperstimulation (COH): the use of fertility drugs to induce a woman's ovaries to produce multiple oocytes during a single cycle

cryopreservation: the storage of live tissue, such as sperm or embryos, by freezing

cul de sac: the area behind the uterus where mature eggs are released by the ovary (also known as the Pouch of Douglas)

cumulus cells: the cells that surround a newly-released oocyte

Demerol: meperidine hydrochloride, a pain-relieving narcotic medication

distal: farther

DNA: deoxyribonucleic acid, the molecules which make up an individual's unique genetic structure and which determine hereditary characteristics

embryo: the initial stage of life, formed just after the egg has been fertilized by the sperm

endometrial biopsy: a diagnostic fertility test in which a portion of the endometrium is removed from the uterus and examined by a pathologist

endometriosis: the condition in which tissue microscopically similar to the uterine lining is found outside of the uterus, on the surfaces of the Fallopian tubes and ovaries

endometrium: the tissue that lines the inside of the uterus

epididymis: the tube-like portion of the male anatomy which extends from the testes. Sperm mature as they swim the length of the epididymis.

epididymitis: inflammation of the epididymis

estradiol: naturally-occurring estrogen

estrogen: the basic female hormone

falloposcope: an instrument that allows the doctor to look inside the Fallopian tubes

Fertinex: an injectable fertility drug consisting of FSH

fibroid: a benign tumor of the uterus

fimbria: finger-like projections at the far ends of the Fallopian tubes

follicle: the ovarian sac (or cyst) in which the oocyte develops

follicle-stimulating hormone (FSH): the hormone that stimulates egg production

follicular puncture: process by which mature follicles are removed from the ovary via a needle which is passed through the rear wall of the vagina

fragment: when parts of an embryo begin to break up

genetic mutation: an alteration in the nature of a gene

gonadotropin: a hormone that acts directly on the ovary to stimulate the production of multiple follicles during a single follicle

granulosa cells: cells that surround the oocyte

hamster egg penetration test: traditional fertility test that evaluates the potential ability of a male's sperm to fertilize a human egg

HCG: human chorionic gonadotropin, the early pregnancy hormone that, in injectable form, acts like LH, causing the final steps of egg development

heparin: a blood thinner

Humegon: an injectable fertility drug consisting of FSH and LH

hydrosalpinx: a condition caused by a prior infection which causes the Fallopian tube to become filled with fluid

hyperthyroidism: the condition in which the thyroid is overly active

hypothalamus: a control center in the brain which governs ovulation by stimulating the pituitary gland

hypothyroidism: the condition in which the thyroid gland is underactive

hysterosalpingogram (HSG): dye-assisted x-ray of the uterus and Fallopian tubes

In vitro: out of the body

In vitro **Fertilization:** procedure in which a woman's eggs are fertilized outside of her body and the resulting embryos are transferred back to her uterus

In vivo: in the body

intracytoplasmic sperm injection (ICSI): the procedure in which a single sperm is injected into an egg to achieve fertilization

Intraperitoneal Insemination (IPI): a procedure in which processed sperm are injected through the rear wall of the vagina into the cul de sac at the time of ovulation

Intrauterine Insemination (IUI): a procedure which calls for processed sperm to be inserted into the top of the woman's uterus

IVIG: intravenous therapy with gamma globulin (mixed blood products)

laparoscopy: a surgical procedure in which a telescope is inserted through a small incision in the woman's abdomen for diagnostic and/or therapeutic purposes

leukocyte: white blood cell

luteal phase defect: inadequate progesterone secretion during the post-ovulatory phase of a woman's menstrual cycle

Luteinized Unruptured Follicle (LUF) Syndrome: condition in which it appears that ovulation has occurred, but the egg is not actually released from the ovary

luteinizing hormone (LH): the hormone which causes the final step of egg maturation

meiosis: the process of reduction division, when the number of chromosomes contained in the egg reduces from 46 to 23

Metaphase II: the name for the stage of egg development that occurs after the number of chromosomes has reduced from 46 to 23

Metrodin: an injectable fertility drug consisting of FSH, not currently being produced. Metrodin was equivalent to Fertinex, but needed to be administered intramuscularly rather than subcutaneously

micromanipulate: to perform procedures on minuscule structures under the microscope

Microsurgical Epididymal Sperm Aspiration (MESA): a procedure to extract sperm from men with obstructions in their epididymal ducts

morphology: shape

morula: the embryonic stage which occurs 4 to 5 days after fertilization and is characterized by a mass of cells within the zona pellucida

motility: movement

mycoplasma: a bacteria-like organism sometimes found in the reproductive tract, that may (or may not) be related to infertility and miscarriage

oocyte: developing egg

Ovarian Hyperstimulation Syndrome (OHSS): condition caused by fertility drugs, in which an unidentified substance causes the fluid component of blood to seep through the walls of the blood vessels into the patient's abdomen or chest cavities

patent: open

Pergonal: an injectable fertility drug consisting of FSH and LH

pituitary gland: the gland responsible for production of the reproductive hormones FSH and LH

polar body: the structure created during fertilization, which contains the extra chromosomal material eliminated by the embryo

Polycystic Ovary Disease (PCO): condition in which the ovary contains numerous, small immature follicular (egg) cysts

polyspermy: condition in which an egg is fertilized by more than one sperm

post-coital test (PCT): test of whether the male's sperm are able to reach and survive in the female's cervical mucus

Pouch of Douglas: the area behind the uterus where mature eggs are released by the ovary (also called the cul de sac)

progesterone: the hormone produced during the second half of the menstrual cycle

prolactin: the hormone responsible for causing milk secretion

pronuclei: a mass of genetic material found inside an egg soon after entry of the sperm

prostatitis: inflammation of the prostate gland

proximal: near

seminal plasma: fluid in the ejaculate

sonogram: an image created through ultrasound technology

spindle mechanism: the mechanism on which the chromosomes of the egg and sperm are arranged for distribution during the course of fertilization

subcutaneous: below the skin

superovulation: the process of using fertility drugs to induce the ovary to produce multiple mature follicles per month

Testicular Extraction of Sperm (TESE): the process which calls for the surgical extraction of small pieces of the testicle for the purpose of harvesting sperm

varicocele: a varicose vein in the scrotum

velocity: speed

Versed: midazolam HCl, a medication used for preoperative sedation

zona pellucida: the outermost layer surrounding the oocyte and, eventually, the embryo

INDEX

acrosome 16, 23, 169

adenomyosis 144-145, 169

age, relevance to fertility 21, 43, 46-47, 128

alcohol 53

anatomy, human vs. rabbit female 11-13

aneuploidy 22, 169

antibodies and infertility, general 146-150, 169
      anticardiolipin antibodies 147
      antichlamydial antibodies 31, 45, 55, 58, 169
      anti-DNA antibodies 147
      antiphospholipids 147
      anti-sperm antibodies 13, 22, 42, 60
      antithyroid antibodies 147

autoimmune diseases 146, 169

basal body temperature (BBT): see also ovulation tests 41, 58, 169

cell division 14-15, 16-17

chlamydia 45, 58, 169

cigarette smoke, effect on fertility 53

Clomid (see clomiphene citrate)

clomiphene citrate 28, 64-67, 156, 169
      as treatment 28, 65
      cost 156
      for diagnostic testing 66
      how it evolved 65
      pros and cons 66-67

co-culture 113-114, 118-119, 169

conception 6-17
      and genetic abnormalities 20-22
      barriers to 20-23
      the odds 20-21

controlled ovarian hyperstimulation (COH) 29, 55, 64-67, 78-82, 91-101, 170
      potential risks 98-101

The Pregnancy Prescription

Too often, infertile couples are treated as medical patients, subject to costly and invasive tests, procedures, and even surgery in an effort to diagnose and then treat whatever is keeping them from conceiving.

But infertility is not a disease. It is the natural process of reproduction gone awry...and conception is far too complex to dissect and repair with any degree of reliability.

The Pregnancy Prescription presents a step-by-step plan for overcoming infertility through the revolutionary, success-oriented approach. By augmenting the natural process of conception and using state-of-the-art advanced reproductive techniques to bypass those stages of the reproductive system that appear most likely to be malfunctioning, the success-oriented approach can help resolve your infertility as quickly, safely, and cost-effectively as possible—no matter where you are in your quest for a pregnancy.

About the Authors

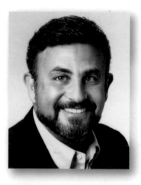

Hugh D. Melnick, M.D., is founder and director of one of the first independent, non-hospital-based infertility centers: Advanced Fertility Services in New York City. He is a leader in the field of infertility treatment and has helped thousands of couples conceive through the success-oriented approach. Dr. Melnick has specialized in infertility and reproductive endocrinology since 1974.

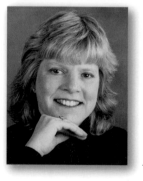

Nancy Intrator is a writer from Chappaqua, NY who specializes in health and family-related topics. Her work has appeared in national publications including American Health, Cosmopolitan, Working Mother, Yachting, The Christian Science Monitor and specialized publications targeted to the health care industry. As a past patient of Dr. Melnick, she successfully conceived using the success-oriented approach.

ISBN 0-9660419-0-9

51795

9 780966 041903

USA $17.95
(Canada $24.95)
Cover Design by Jane Birkenstock

THE JOSARA COMPANIES, INC.

*For the staff of Advanced Fertility Services,
without whose efforts none of this
would have been possible. — H.M.*

For Richard, who has always believed in me. — N.I.

TABLE OF CONTENTS

PART III: OTHER CONSIDERATIONS

PART IV: THE ULTIMATE DECISION

PREFACE

Hugh Melnick, MD

If you are reading this book, chances are good that you have traveled a difficult road in your quest to have a baby. You are probably disappointed, frustrated, and afraid that you may never succeed in conceiving the child that you want so badly. You may not know which—if any—of the modern fertility treatments you should try, or whether you are justified in considering yourself "desperate" enough to resort to the new, high-tech approaches. If there are no obvious causes for your failure to conceive, or if you have conceived in the past and now find yourself unable to become pregnant, you are probably just that much more confused.

We wrote this book, *The Pregnancy Prescription,* to help you find your way through the maze of infertility treatments towards the quickest, safest, and most cost-effective path to conception.

But first I had to challenge a few prevalent beliefs.

One notion that needs debunking is that it should be possible for doctors to be able to pinpoint and resolve whatever disorder is preventing a couple from conceiving. I believe that infertility is the failure of a natural process, rather than a "disease" to be diagnosed and treated, and it is my opinion that infertility treatment should be aimed at resolving the symptom—the inability to conceive—rather than by "fixing" whatever is going wrong. In my many years of clinical practice, I have found that conception is just too complex a process to dissect and repair. Instead, I have helped countless couples conceive by augmenting the natural process of conception and, where appropriate, bypassing whatever stage in the process appears, most likely, to be going awry.

I am also compelled to dispute the myth that people with infertility are somehow responsible for their own inability to conceive. For instance, one current theory is that one or both members of a couple harbor some unknown psychological barrier to parenthood deep within their subconscious, and that these thoughts are subverting their conscious efforts to become pregnant. On another level, infertile couples often believe that they have caused the problem themselves, due to some "fatal error" like having had intercourse one day too early or late, or by the woman not having spent enough time lying in bed with her legs up after sex. I do not believe in either of these possibilities. Perhaps the most important lesson I have learned in more than twenty years of working with infertile couples is that even with all the scientific advances we have achieved, conception is largely beyond human control. In my experience, nature only allows those embryos that are most likely to become healthy, perfect babies to develop and implant. If we accept this and trust in nature, we can better accept the pain and frustration of infertility.

The Pregnancy Prescription will provide you with an individualized roadmap to help you find your way through the labyrinth of infertility. By guiding you toward the most direct route possible given your unique reproductive characteristics, I hope to make your journey to conception both quick and successful.

Hugh Melnick, MD

PREFACE

Nancy Intrator

In 1985 my husband and I had our first child, Joshua. Josh was conceived "the old-fashioned way," with the help of a few dimly lit candles and a bottle of fine wine. His conception was well-planned. When Richard and I married in 1974, we had agreed to wait ten years before having our first baby. Newly graduated from college, we had careers to launch, trips to take, empty bank accounts to fill, and all the time in the world—or so we thought.

Our little boy was a constant delight, and when he was two we decided it was time for another. Only this time, it wasn't so easy. First we tried on our own, then we tried with some help from my OB/GYN, and finally, the doctor advised us to see Dr. Hugh Melnick if we wanted to keep on trying. We resisted the thought of a fertility specialist; I had, after all, conceived once on my own. But I was already 38, and I really, *really* wanted another baby.

On my first visit to Advanced Fertility Services in New York City, I immediately felt as though I was in the right place. The staff seemed to truly care about their patients. The atmosphere was warm and enveloping, like a big bear hug. And when I met Dr. Melnick, I finally allowed myself to feel hopeful that I might someday conceive the second child I longed for.

"I won't give up on you," he promised.

And he didn't. During the time we worked together, as the technology for infertility treatment advanced, so too did the forms of my treatment. With the help of Dr. Melnick and his staff,

I made my way through inseminations, injections, x-rays, and IVF. Finally, in 1992, I gave birth to my beautiful daughter, Sara.

Dr. Melnick and I formed a lasting friendship during my fertility treatment. I've had the privilege of seeing countless couples have their dreams of pregnancy come true, thanks to Hugh Melnick. And because we both believe so strongly in his success-oriented approach, we decided to make his vision accessible to infertile couples everywhere, through this book: *The Pregnancy Prescription.*

Although the book is primarily in the voice of Hugh Melnick, please know that it comes also from one who understands how it feels to want a baby more than anything else in the world.

Nancy Intrator

ACKNOWLEDGEMENTS

My deepest thanks go to my co-author, Nancy Intrator, for making the writing of this book a totally enjoyable experience.

My appreciation goes also to Carolyn Menna for her insightful editorial assistance and to Marc S. Cohen, MD, for his contributions in the areas of urology and andrology.

Special thanks to my son, Josh Melnick and to Kent Thanki, PhD, Chief Embryologist at Advanced Fertility Services, for their help in creating photographs for this book.

I would also like to express my eternal gratitude to my mentors, Hugh R.K. Barber, MD, the late Herbert S. Kupperman, MD, PhD, Herman Friedman, PhD, and my parents, Everett and Selma, who were all a great source of inspiration for my professional endeavors.

H.M.

Acknowledgements

Thanks to Candy Schulman for her invaluable assistance in shaping this book and for helping me find my voice as a writer.

Many thanks to Carol Ross for her patience and generosity in answering my endless questions about the publishing industry.

Our sincere appreciation to Kathryn Pucci for her editorial talents and to Ray Mara for his guidance throughout the production process.

My heartfelt appreciation to the past and present members of my writer's group, whose support, encouragement, and gentle criticism sustained me throughout this project.

A loving "thank you" to my children, Josh and Sara, who never complained when I responded to their requests for meals, attention, etc. with the inevitable "Just let me finish this page."

Finally, my everlasting gratitude to my very dear friend, Dr. Hugh Melnick, who helped make it possible for two of my fondest wishes to come true.

N.I.

THE
PREGNANCY
PRESCRIPTION

The
Success-Oriented
Approach to
Overcoming Infertility

INTRODUCTION

THE SUCCESS-ORIENTED STRATEGY FOR OVERCOMING INFERTILITY

IS THIS YOU?

I want a baby more than anything else in the world.

Surely this will be the month, I tell myself at the beginning of each cycle. But then somewhere around day nine, the panic sets in. Will sperm and egg be available when they're needed? Could they possibly manage to meet up in the right place, at the right time, just this once? Will even a single solitary sperm make the effort to poke itself deeply enough inside the egg to make it fertilize?

For us, sex has nothing to do with love anymore. With all the timing and planning, it's gotten to feel like more of a chore than anything else.

The last two weeks of each month are the hardest. Either a potential new life has begun—or not. The outcome has been determined; all we can do is wait and wonder.

At the end of the month, I deny the physical signs of my impending period until the flow begins, proving that once again, I have not conceived.

We've gone through so many tests and treatments. None of them seem to have gotten us any closer to having a baby.

I've never before felt such a complete loss of control.

INFERTILITY AFFECTS EVERY PART OF YOU

If you've been through even 1 month of unsuccessfully trying to conceive, you are only too well aware of the enormous effect infertility can have on every aspect of your life. It can wreak havoc on your emotions. It can change the way you feel about yourself, your partner, and your relationships. It can affect the way you do your job. It can deplete your financial reserves. It can destroy your faith.

But few infertility patients are "lucky" enough to go through all this for only 1 month. The more likely scenario is that an infertile couple will spend countless months—or even years—trying for a pregnancy. Their doctor may find a few possible explanations for their infertility and try to fix whatever is wrong, but too often, the couple ends up no closer to realizing their dream. They don't know *why* they're not succeeding—and frankly, they don't really care. They just know that they want to conceive a baby...as *quickly, safely,* and *cost-effectively* as possible.

THE PREGNANCY PRESCRIPTION

The Pregnancy Prescription will show you a more direct route to conception. This success-oriented approach calls for using state-of-the-art reproductive technology to *bypass* whatever problems may be keeping you from becoming pregnant, instead of counseling you to waste precious time, energy, and money trying to diagnose and resolve those problems. If you haven't been able to conceive on your own after trying for a reasonable amount of time, there's a good chance that your problems would eventually prove impossible to diagnose and/or resolve anyway.

Although no infertility treatment can be guaranteed to make you pregnant, the strategy described in this book represents a medically sound, highly effective, efficient, safe, and cost-effective alternative to the traditional diagnosis- and treatment-oriented approach.

WHERE DO I BEGIN?

Depending on where you are in your quest for a child, you may need to begin following *The Pregnancy Prescription* at different stages. The following are some suggestions on where to start:

IF YOU OR YOUR PARTNER	BEGIN AT
are just beginning to worry about infertility	chapter 1
feel as though you may have caused your infertility by something you have or haven't done correctly	chapter 2
are just selecting your infertility doctor	chapter 3
are about to begin diagnostic testing	chapter 4
have irregular menstrual cycles, an abnormal sperm count, or unexplained infertility	chapter 5
have not conceived with oral fertility drugs and intrauterine insemination	chapter 6

have not conceived after numerous
cycles with insemination and fertility drugs

or have blocked Fallopian tubes or an extremely
poor sperm count

or test positive for antichlamydial antibodies

or have had longstanding (3 to 4 years) infertility   chapter 7

have been told that your eggs may have
begun to deteriorate   chapter 8

are considering IVF with donor eggs   chapter 9

are concerned that there might be some
undiagnosed problem with your uterus   chapter 10

are worried about the cost of treatment   chapter 11

HOW THIS BOOK CAN HELP

By increasing your awareness of all possible options at each step, *The Pregnancy Prescription* can provide a roadmap for helping you plot the most direct route to resolving your infertility. Its success-oriented strategy can help you regain control over your reproductive life...and it just might make it possible for your dream of a pregnancy to come true.

CHAPTER 1

NATURAL REPRODUCTION:

How The Process Should Work

If you are trying to have a baby, chances are good that you already understand the basics of reproduction. What you may not realize is that conception is like a game of dominoes: if all the pieces are in perfect alignment, each will fall in its proper sequence until none are left standing. But if even just one single piece is slightly out of line, the whole process will fail.

This quick review of oocyte development, fertilization, and implantation may help you better understand some of the factors that might be working against you.

OOCYTE DEVELOPMENT

A woman's menstrual cycle is the result of an elegant system of hormonal signals that is self-programmed to produce a mature, chromosomally and genetically appropriate egg, each cycle.

A Lifetime Supply

A baby girl is born with all the eggs she will ever have in her life-time. These eggs, which usually number about 500,000, develop while the fetus is still in the mother's uterus, and then remain in a resting state in the ovaries until the girl reaches puberty at about 11 to14 years of age. Once she begins menstruating, approxi-mately 1,000 of her eggs will become stimulated each month. Of these, only one (or rarely, two) will become mature and be released from the ovary each month. The rest regress and die. On average, a woman's lifetime supply of eggs will be diminished by approximately 12,000 per year, and over a 30-year period, she may lose as many as 360,000 of the original 500,000.

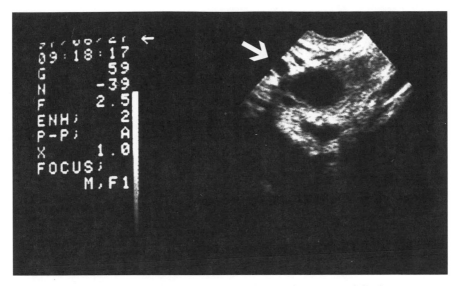

Fig. 1. *Sonogram showing the ovary with a single mature follicle, which contains a single egg inside.*

The Hormones That Help Eggs Grow

The key hormones responsible for egg development are estrogen (the primary female hormone), follicle-stimulating hormone (FSH), and luteinizing hormone (LH). Both FSH and LH are produced by the pituitary gland as a result of stimulation from the hypothalamus, a control center in the brain, while estrogen is produced by the cells that surround the egg in the ovary.

At the beginning of a woman's menstrual cycle, her eggs and the "granulosa" cells which surround them are in a resting state, so her estrogen levels are quite low. The brain's control center senses this low estrogen level and stimulates the pituitary gland to begin producing FSH. The FSH causes an egg to begin maturing and stimulates the granulosa cells surrounding that egg to begin producing estrogen. As her estrogen level rises, the amount of FSH produced by the woman's pituitary gland begins to fall.

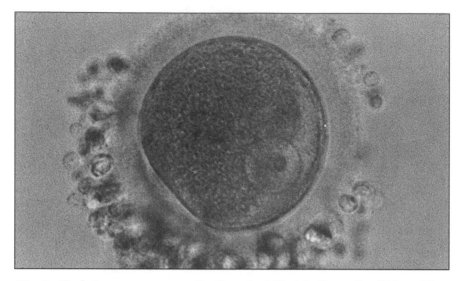

Fig. 2. *Early immature egg at the Germinal Vessicle Stage. It still has 46 chromosomes and has not yet undergone reduction division to the mature egg status of 23 chromosomes.*

Once an ovarian follicle starts being stimulated, it becomes the "dominant follicle" and begins growing approximately 2 millimeters (mm) per day. The egg is considered to be in the fertile zone when the follicle measures 20 mm, which is slightly less than 1 inch. Although the mature egg itself is microscopic (approximately 100 mature eggs will fit on the head of a pin) the growth of the follicle—the ovarian sac in which the egg grows— can be tracked through ultrasound.

Final Steps to Maturity

When the woman's estrogen level reaches a critically high point, it provides a sign that the egg is near maturity. This triggers a different center in the brain to stimulate the pituitary gland to release vast stores of LH, which causes the final step of egg maturation. In this final stage, called reduction division (meiosis), the number of chromosomes contained in the egg reduces from 46 (normal humans have 46 chromosomes per cell) to 23. Since there are 23 chromosomes in a mature, normal sperm cell, when sperm and egg are united through fertilization, the resulting embryo should come into possession of its full complement of 46 chromosomes: 23 from the biological mother via the egg, and 23 from the biological father, through the sperm.

Frequently, too much genetic material may be transferred to the embryo. This can be caused by failure in the reduction division stage of the oocyte or by the egg being fertilized by two sperm at once (polyspermy). When this happens, the pregnancy is defective and will usually result in miscarriage. In fact, genetic errors are the most common causes of miscarriage.

OOCYTE RELEASE

Approximately 36 hours after the LH surge, the follicle in which the egg is contained will burst. The egg is released, along with its

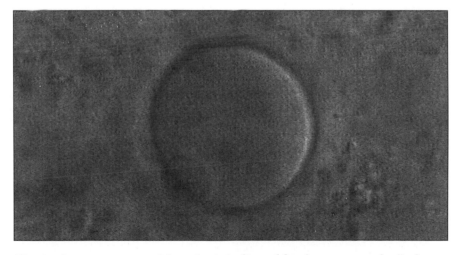

Fig. 3. *A mature oocyte. Maturity is indicated by the presence of a "polar body", the round structure found at the edge of the egg in the 7 o'clock position. This polar body contains the 23 chromosomes which have been discarded as a result of reduction division. This is the end point of egg maturity.*

surrounding granulosa cells and the follicular fluid, which contains a variety of proteins and hormones.

It is truly remarkable that the final steps of egg maturation (meiosis) and the ultimate release of the mature egg are both governed by the same hormone, LH. This is nature's way of ensuring that a fully matured egg, with the appropriate genetic constitution, will be released at the appropriate time each month.

FERTILIZATION

Survival of the Fittest

The high levels of estrogen that help to signal the LH surge and bring about the release of the egg also serve to increase the quality and quantity of mucus in the woman's cervix, uterus, and Fallopian tubes. The mucus acts as a preservative for the sperm that are ejaculated into the vagina and helps filter out abnormal sperm.

When the man ejaculates, only 10% of his sperm actually makes it to the cervical mucus. The rest perish in the vagina which, due to its acidity, is not well-suited to supporting their longevity. From that point on, "survival of the fittest" is the rule: the farther up through the genital tract the sperm travel, the fewer survive. In fact, some studies have shown that even if as many as 100-200 million sperm have been ejaculated into a woman's vagina, only 500 live sperm may arrive in each of her Fallopian tubes. Those that do reach their ultimate destination are not only the strongest, but also the fastest: studies have shown that sperm may arrive at the outer ends of the Fallopian tubes as early as 10 minutes after insemination.

Early is Better Than Late

Since sperm have been proven capable of surviving as long as 5 to7 days in a mucus-lined genital tract or uterine cavity, the precise timing of intercourse is not critical for fertilization. This should help reduce the psychological pressure for couples who believe it is necessary to achieve split-second accuracy in the timing of intercourse. Recent studies indicate, though, that pregnancy is most likely to occur when intercourse takes place in the period just before the egg has been released. Cervical mucus can start to become hostile to sperm beginning at about 18 hours after the egg has been released (or 54 to 58 hours after the LH surge), and once that has happened, the sperm can no longer survive.

Where Egg Meets Sperm

In certain species, the female anatomy seems designed to help increase the chances for fertilization and conception. In female rabbits, the Fallopian tube surrounds the ovary. When the rabbit releases her eggs, they are deposited directly into the Fallopian tube, where fertilization takes place. This anatomical advantage is a likely explanation for why rabbits are so fertile and how the phrase "multiply like rabbits" was coined.

But a human female is built quite differently than a female rabbit. The tiny (<1 mm) opening of a human Fallopian tube lies at least 4 to 6 centimeters (1.5 to 2.5 inches) away from its source of eggs. It is anatomically impossible for a human egg to be caught by the Fallopian tube as it is released from the ovary.

So how does it get there?

Our theory is that after the follicle ruptures, the egg and follicular fluid accumulate in a pool in the area behind the uterus

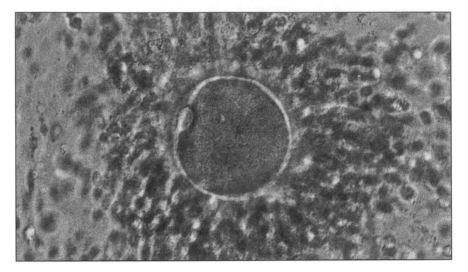

Fig. 4. *Egg cumulus as it appears when it first emerges from the ovary.*

known as the Pouch of Douglas (or cul de sac). Since sperm that successfully travel to the ends of the Fallopian tubes are also found in the Pouch of Douglas, we believe that this may be where the egg and sperm unite. The sticky, finger-like projections at the ends of the Fallopian tubes, called fimbria, dip into this pool.

When eggs are manually removed from the ovary during *In Vitro* Fertilization (IVF), they are surrounded by sticky, cumulus cells. We believe that an attachment takes place between the fimbria and these cumulus cells, and that the fimbria actually suck the egg/cumulus structure out of the cul de sac and into the opening of the tube either through very fine muscular contractions or via propulsion by the cilia (hairlike cells) that line the female genital tract.

At Advanced Fertility Services in New York City, we have developed a procedure called Intraperitoneal Insemination (IPI), in which we inject small numbers of sperm through the wall of the vagina and into the cul de sac fluid soon after ovulation has taken place. This technique, which has been in use since 1986, has resulted in pregnancies for a number of women who were unable to conceive via normal intrauterine insemination. This may be because the sperm are placed directly into the area where the eggs have been deposited, making it easier for them to come into direct contact with the egg. Or, the process may protect the sperm from anti-sperm antibodies or other toxic substances that may be secreted by the uterus or circulated through the Fallopian tubes. Intraperitoneal Insemination is described in greater detail in Chapter 6.

Becoming an Embryo

When sperm and egg meet during the initial stages of fertilization, hundreds of sperm may attempt to penetrate the thick layers of granulosa cells that surround the egg. Those sperm that swim with a strong enough velocity will latch onto receptors on the surface of the egg, similar to the way a spaceship latches onto

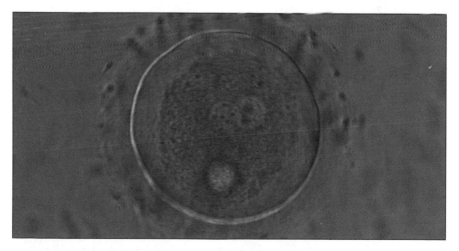

Fig. 5. *An early embryo, 18 hours after fertilization with many sperm bound to its surface. Two pronuclei are present in the center of the newly-formed embryo.*

EMBRYOS

Fig. 6. *Earliest stage of embryo — the 2 pronuclear stage. 18 hours after fertilization the two round structures in the center of the egg indicate that a single sperm has penetrated the egg successfully.*

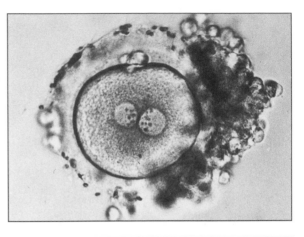

Fig. 7. *The embryo divides into two cells after twenty-four hours. Each cell, called a blastomere, will continue to split and cause an increase in the number of cells contained within the walls of the zona pellucida.*

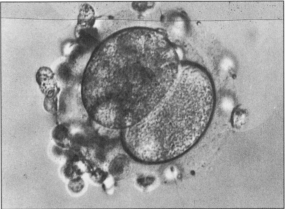

Fig. 8. *An embryo should be at the four cell stage 48 hours after fertilization.*

A four cell embryo at 48 hours.

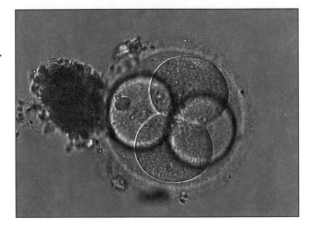

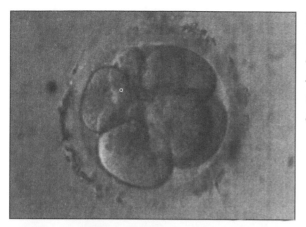

Fig. 9. *A six cell embryo is an intermediate step and may either indicate slow development or an unequal rate of cell division.*

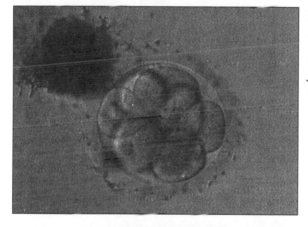

Fig. 10. *An eight cell embryo should be present by 72 hours post fertilization at the time of embryo transfer.*

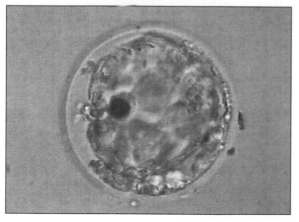

Fig. 11. *An expanded blastocyst after six days in the incubator.*

a landing site on a space station. After a sperm has locked on, a reaction begins that causes it to release a package of enzymes (the acrosome) located in the head of the sperm, to help it penetrate the outer shell of the egg, which is known as the zona pellucida.

Once the first sperm has successfully penetrated the shell, no other sperm will likely gain entry. If an egg were to become fertilized by more than one sperm (polyspermia), the resulting embryo would contain more than the normal amount of genetic material, making it incapable of surviving. Embryos created as a result of polyspermy are always destined to miscarry at a very early stage of development.

If there has been successful fertilization, two pronuclei (round, circular structures) will be visible inside the egg approximately eighteen hours later. One of these circular structures contains genetic material from the egg, (23 chromosomes), and the other holds the same amount of genetic material from the sperm. The two pronuclei then break down and fuse, providing the embryo with its full complement of 46 chromosomes.

Once the pronuclei have broken down, the embryo begins to divide. Approximately 48 hours after fertilization the embryo will consist of 2 to 4 cells; by 72 hours post-fertilization, there will be 6 to 8 cells. At that point, cell division begins to occur rapidly. By 4 to 5 days after fertilization, the embryo will consist of more than 60 cells within the zona pellucida. This is called the morula stage.

Implantation

As cell division occurs, the embryo makes its way from the fimbria through the length of the Fallopian tube and into the uterus. By the time it has reached its destination, the embryo is in the blastocyst stage, at which time the zona pellucida breaks down and the embryo "hatches," or bursts out of its shell. Hatching is critical, because the shell limits the ability of the embryo to expand and prevents it from implanting into the lining of the uterus. Implantation usually occurs 5 to 7 days after fertilization.

SUMMARY

The human reproductive system is set up in a very logical, almost foolproof manner so that we should be equipped to reproduce quite efficiently. But even a single, minor glitch in the process can interrupt an entire cycle and prevent the ultimate objective, which is the fertilization of the egg by the sperm. In Chapter 2, you will learn more about these "glitches," and how they may be sabotaging you in your struggle to conceive.

BARRIERS TO CONCEPTION:

What Could Be Going Wrong?

T he first thing that you and your partner need to understand *and believe* is that your inability to conceive has nothing to do with anything that either of you has or hasn't done. You could not have "ruined" a potential pregnancy by jogging during the last half of your cycle or subjecting yourself to too much stress on the job. Most embryos miscarry due to genetic abnormalities that are present either in the chromosome content or in the individual genes located on the chromosomes. Such factors that are completely beyond your—or anyone's—control.

THE ODDS

Since each and every one of our chromosome carries thousands of different genes, the potential for genetic abnormality in a newly created embryo is huge. Nature doesn't allow the vast majority of embryos with chromosomal or genetic abnormalities to survive to the point that would make a woman's period late or give her a positive pregnancy test. Instead, these embryos self-destruct in a natural, fail-safe mechanism that prevents the birth of abnormal babies.

It is important to realize that the vast majority of every woman's eggs probably contains genetic mutations. It is impossible to test for these mutations because of the tremendous number of genes present: each of the 23 chromosomes in a mature egg (or sperm) has thousands of gene sites on it, each with a unique, complex molecular structure. This is why, even if all of the steps leading to fertilization and implantation take place perfectly, *any* embryo still has only a 20 percent chance of developing into a clinically observable pregnancy.

Although nature causes approximately 80 percent of potential embryos to "miscarry" before a pregnancy becomes evident, the 20% that are left cannot all be considered sound. An additional 25 to 35 percent may hang on long enough to cause a positive pregnancy test, but will prove incapable of surviving longer than 6 to 8 weeks.

Once a fetal heartbeat can be detected, the prospective parents can breathe easier. At that point, the chance of miscarriage declines from 35 to 5 percent.

WHAT'S AGE GOT TO DO WITH IT?

Even prior to birth, a woman's eggs lie dormant in her ovaries. Her genetic material, the DNA found on the chromosomes, remains in a resting state. As time passes and the woman ages, the electrical charges that hold the DNA molecules together may become weaker and less able to maintain the DNA in the exact shape and configuration necessary for the creation of a structurally perfect offspring. These alterations, known as genetic mutations, are probably among the leading causes of miscarriage and may be responsible for the reduction in fertility experienced by women as they grow older.

In comparison to the woman's eggs, sperm have an extremely short (72 to 96 days) life cycle. This means that the DNA contained within any individual sperm can be no more than two-to-three months old at any time, and the electrochemical bonds that hold sperm DNA in position are less likely to deteriorate.

MORE GENETIC MAYHEM

Abnormal chromosome distribution, which can begin just prior to fertilization, is another common cause of genetic mishap which results in a condition called aneuploidy. An aneuploidic embryo has either too much or too little genetic information.

At the time of fertilization, the chromosomes belonging to both the egg and the sperm are arranged for distribution on a spindle mechanism. If the spindle fails to operate correctly, this will cause the embryo to be left with either too many or too few chromosomes. In most cases, having too many or too few chromosomes is "lethal" for an embryo and will result in a very early miscarriage.

AS IF THAT WEREN'T ENOUGH...

In addition to genetic abnormalities, there are many other factors that can prevent conception:

For The Woman

- Hormonal imbalances may prevent the woman from producing a viable egg
- The uterine lining may not develop well enough to become capable of sustaining a pregnancy
- The woman may have fibroids or some other uterine abnormality that prevents the embryo from implanting
- The woman's cervical mucus may be hostile to her partner's sperm (either due to infection or an antibody reaction)
- The woman's eggs may not be able to be fertilized
- The woman's Fallopian tubes may be blocked, preventing access to the eggs by the sperm

- The Fallopian tubes may not function properly in picking up or transporting the eggs

For The Man

- Too few sperm may be produced

- The motility (movement) of the sperm may be insufficient to move the sperm from the vagina to the cervix, or beyond that to the Fallopian tubes

- The sperm may not have receptors to enable it to bind to an egg

- The sperm may not have the enzymes (acrosome) to "eat" its way into the egg

- The sperm may not have the velocity (speed, or energy) to penetrate cumulus cells surrounding the egg

- The sperm may contain abnormal genetic material

SUMMARY

There are many possible reasons why you may not be conceiving. Genetic abnormalities are so common that, even if all the steps in the conception process are perfectly aligned, pregnancy will not be produced in the majority of cycles. But unless there is an *obvious* problem—such as blocked Fallopian tubes—it may be impossible to pinpoint exactly where the problem may lie.

The Pregnancy Prescription can offer you a new perspective on your infertility situation...even if whatever is preventing you from conceiving turns out to be impossible to diagnose or treat.

CHAPTER 3

APPROACHES TO INFERTILITY TREATMENT:

Success-Oriented vs. Diagnosis-Oriented

Any infertility specialist will want to help you conceive a child, but they all won't necessarily go about it in the same way. The difference will lie in the diagnostic tests they order, the procedures they recommend, and in their overall goals for your treatment.

In general, infertility specialists can be considered either "diagnosis-oriented" or "success-oriented." Here, in a nutshell, are the differences between the two approaches:

	SUCCESS-ORIENTED APPROACH	TRADITIONAL DIAGNOSIS-AND-TREATMENT APPROACH
Diagnosis	A few, limited tests to identify problem steps. Should take only a few cycles and cost approximately $1,500.	Extensive diagnostic workup that may take more than one year to perform and cost up to $9,000.
Treatment	Augment nature or bypass problem steps.	Resolve diagnosed disorders and then try for natural conception. Repeat process as many times as necessary.
In Vitro **Fertilization**	Used early in the process for diagnosis *and* treatment.	Used as last-resort treatment option.

THE TRADITIONAL, DIAGNOSIS-ORIENTED APPROACH

Although diagnosis-oriented physicians agree that pregnancy is the ultimate goal for their patients, their primary objectives are first, to diagnose the cause of the couple's infertility, and then to try and resolve the problem(s). Theoretically, this should enable the couple to go on to conceive naturally.

Diagnosis-oriented physicians treat infertility like a disease. They use exhaustive tests and procedures to try and determine exactly which element in a couple's reproductive process is not working correctly. If the results of any of these tests signal a problem, the diagnosis-oriented physician will treat whatever problem is found. The couple will probably go on to spend several months trying to conceive on their own. If the identified problem turned out to be the only factor standing in the way of conception, the couple will probably conceive fairly quickly. But if the woman is still unable to become pregnant, it could mean that either the diagnosis was incorrect, the treatment was ineffective, or there is more than one problem keeping her from conceiving.

The majority of diagnosis-oriented physicians believe that advanced reproductive techniques such as IVF are treatment tools to be used only after all attempts to diagnose and correct the source of the problem have failed to help the couple conceive. In their opinion, IVF is the "court of last resort."

THE MODERN, SUCCESS-ORIENTED APPROACH

Success-oriented physicians believe that conception is the single most important goal of infertility treatment. These doctors feel that the best way to help an infertile couple is to perform only those diagnostic tests that will identify the steps in the reproductive process that are most likely to be causing the problem, and then to use the available technology to bypass those steps. This is because these physicians believe that infertility is not a disease, but rather a biological malfunction that occurs in perfectly healthy individuals. Since the kinds of problems that cause infertility have no other negative effect on a person's overall health or well-being, success-oriented physicians believe that a diagnosis-oriented approach will not be as effective in resolving infertility as it is in treating true illnesses or injuries.

The main steps in the success-oriented approach, as described in *The Pregnancy Prescription,* are:

Step 1: The Streamlined Workup. An abbreviated diagnostic workup is used to determine whether the couple is potentially fertile, and to identify the steps that are most likely to be preventing them from conceiving.

Step 2: Clomiphene citrate and Intrauterine Insemination (IUI). The oral fertility drug, clomiphene citrate (brand names Clomid™, Serophene™) is used to increase the number of eggs the woman is able to produce. Intrauterine insemination, which calls for a specially prepared sperm specimen to be inserted into the top of the woman's uterus, provides the sperm with direct access to the Fallopian tubes, bypassing possible problems in the vagina and cervix.

Step 3: Gonadotropins and Intraperitoneal Insemination (IPI). Injectable fertility drugs (gonadotropins: Pergonal™, Humegon™, Fertinex™, Follistim™, and Gonal F™) induce the woman to produce far greater numbers of mature eggs (controlled ovarian hyperstimulation) than the oral fertility medication used in Step 2. IPI (which calls for the processed sperm to be injected through the rear wall of the vagina into the cul de sac while it contains newly-released eggs) brings the sperm even closer to the increased numbers of eggs than is possible with IUI.

Step 4: In vitro Fertilization (IVF). In IVF, the eggs are removed from the ovary and fertilized in the laboratory, away from any potentially detrimental factors within the woman's body. Resulting embryos are placed back into the uterus. The embryologist may use Intracytoplasmic Sperm Injection (ICSI), in which a single sperm is injected into the egg, to help the fertilization process along.

Step 5: IVF With Donor Eggs. When the woman's egg supply is found to be either depleted or unable to be fertilized, her partner's sperm may be used to fertilize donor eggs. The resulting embryos are placed back into the woman's uterus and, should she become pregnant, the baby will be her biological—if not genetic—offspring.

Many of the therapeutic tools used by success-oriented physicians (such as controlled ovarian hyperstimulation with fertility drugs or IVF) also happen to be very effective diagnostic tools for evaluating unexplained infertility. The fact that many of its interventions can both diagnose and treat at the same time makes the success-oriented strategy both efficient and cost-effective.

Former infertility patients confirm that the success-oriented approach is much easier on the emotions, too. From a patient's point of view, any time not spent in the direct pursuit of pregnancy is time wasted. Months lost to testing, aimless "trying," and prescribed time off can cause unspeakable anguish to the woman who wants nothing more than a new life in her belly. The beauty of the success-oriented approach is that conception is possible even during most diagnostic cycles.

Although success-oriented physicians don't believe that all advanced reproductive techniques (like IVF) are right for each and every patient, they do believe that, for many couples, IVF can increase a couple's chance of conceiving *more quickly and cost-effectively* by:

- **Eliminating** the need for some of the more expensive, invasive, and time-consuming diagnostic tests

- **Identifying** non-obvious or undetectable problems that are most likely to be preventing the couple from conceiving

- **Bypassing** the steps that appear most likely to be causing the couple's infertility

- **Offering a 20 percent chance of conception every time it is performed** by bringing egg and sperm together in an environment that provides optimum conditions for fertilization

SUCCESS STORIES

Here are some examples of how the success-oriented approach helped two couples with problems that weren't so easy to detect.

Susan and Mark—The Success-Oriented Approach

Susan and Mark, both 36-year-old lawyers, had been unsuccessfully trying to conceive on their own for 6 months. Susan had an early, uncomplicated abortion before she met Mark, and the couple had been lax about practicing birth control for the several years before they started trying for a pregnancy.

Although nothing suspicious was noted during her case history, Susan's blood tested positive for anti-chlamydial antibodies, indicating that she had previously been infected by that organism.

Because he suspected that Susan's tubes might have been damaged as a result of the infection, the doctor recommended that Susan undergo a hysterosalpingogram (HSG: x-ray of the uterus and Fallopian tubes) as her next step. The x-ray showed that one tube was completely blocked, and the other was open.

Since Susan had tested positive for a previous chlamydia infection, had been unable to become pregnant on her own, and was known to have at least one damaged tube, the doctor suspected that the other tube might have been compromised as well. Taking Susan's age into account, he recommended that the couple proceed directly to an IVF cycle, which would both bypass the tubes and enable the doctor to determine whether there might also be a fertilization problem or some other issue with Mark's sperm.

With the help of medication, Susan produced six eggs for the IVF cycle—four of which were successfully fertilized by Mark's sperm. Although the couple elected to have all four embryos transferred back into Susan's uterus, she did not conceive during that cycle. Since they had achieved good fertilization, the doctor encouraged Susan and Mark to try IVF a few more times. Happily, Susan became pregnant on their second try.

Susan and Mark—The Diagnosis-Oriented Approach

Let's see what could have happened if Susan and Mark had consulted a diagnosis-oriented fertility specialist.

The results of the cervical cultures normally performed during a standard workup would have been negative for Susan, since she suffered from no current chlamydial infection. Therefore, unless the doctor performed a blood test for anti-chlamydial antibodies, he might not have thought to have Susan undergo a hysterosalpingogram (HSG) so early in the diagnostic process. Instead, he might have sent her home with urine testing kits to monitor her ovulation and instructions as to how to schedule intercourse for the appropriate time after the LH surge. At the same time, Mark would have been asked to undergo a semen analysis, the results of which would be normal.

After a few cycles of supposedly normal ovulation but no resulting conception, the doctor would then have been likely to suggest an HSG. Although the x-rays would have shown a blockage in one tube, the doctor would probably have assumed that the other tube was healthy and might have recommended that Susan keep trying to conceive on her own, with the possible assistance of some oral fertility medication. But six months later, when Susan still wasn't pregnant, he might have changed his mind. The doctor might have performed a laparoscopy, using surgery both to repair the known blockage and to look for endometriosis or some other anatomical problem that might be keeping Susan from conceiving. Although the operation would be performed on an outpatient basis, Susan would still need to undergo general anesthesia during the procedure, and she would experience pain and soreness for some time afterward. In addition to having to pay the cost of the surgery, she would also need to skip at least a few days of work while she recovered.

After her laparoscopy, Susan (her damaged tube newly unblocked) and Mark would be ready to try again. This time, the doctor might help things along with both injectable fertility drugs and inseminations. Unfortunately, Susan still would not